IN THE SHADOW OF

VENUS

ALSO BY JOHN POTTERAT

SEEKING THE POSITIVES:
A LIFE SPENT ON THE CUTTING EDGE OF PUBLIC HEALTH

IN THE SHADOW OF VENUS

Vignettes from the Venereal World

Edited By

John J. Potterat

Nancy E. Spencer

Stephen Q. Muth

CREATESPACE
4900 Lacross Rd., North Charleston, SC 29406, U.S.A.
A DBA of On-Demand Publishing, LLC

Copyright © 2017
by John J. Potterat, Nancy E. Spencer & Stephen Q. Muth
All rights reserved, including the right of reproduction
in whole or in part or in any form

Library of Congress Cataloging-in-Publication Data

Potterat, John J.
Spencer, Nancy E.
Muth, Stephen Q.

In The Shadow of Venus
Vignettes from the Venereal World

Includes Index of Vignette Titles
1. Epidemiology – Popular Works
2. Sexually Transmitted Disease – United States
I. Title

ISBN-10: 1976200172
ISBN-13: 978-1976200175

Layout and photography by Stephen Q. Muth, including back cover image of Venus transiting the Sun on 5 June 2012

Sketches, including cover illustration, by N. Fenton

To our patients, who nourished the closet anthropologist in us

"Life is a tragedy when seen in close-up,
but a comedy in long-shot"

—Charlie Chaplin

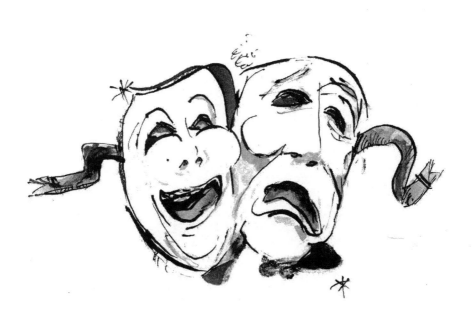

CONTENTS

	Preface	XIII
	Acknowledgment	XIX
Part I:	In Clinic	1
Part II:	Contact Interviewing	31
Part III:	In the Field	61
Part IV:	HIV/AIDS	109
Part V:	Prostitution	157
Part VI:	Behind The Scenes	187
	Contributors	219
	Title Index	225

Preface

> "We have to change the truth a little in order to remember it."
>
> —Santayana

Venus, goddess of love and beauty is also, along with her son Eros, a metaphor for sexual love. And just as a lovely rose has thorns, Venus has a thorny, shadowy side. In its sexual form, love may cause emotional distress, not to mention produce untoward outcomes, whether undesired pregnancy or serious infection. As you're about to see.

This is a book of anecdotes by professionals doing venereal disease (VD) control, about people met on the VD front lines, and for people who are curious about this unusual, exotic line of work. Virtually all take place in Colorado during the last thirty years of the 20th century. But don't let this provincial locale fool you: in these particular anecdotes lie universal experiences, irrespective of geography or time.

It's not possible to spend years, nay decades, striving to control venereal (from "Venus") infections and fail to see human foibles in a starkly naked way.

Routinely asking infected people the supremely private questions one must ask—with whom they have sex, in what ways, how often, and where—is key to elucidating, and thus eventually controlling, venereal disease propagation.

Through these brief vignettes you'll be introduced not simply to some of the various people encountered but also to yourself. For how many of us have not been—or could have been—in similar circumstances? The vignettes are intended to act as a mirror of human nature, with empathy sharpening what's being observed. It's also good to remember that mirrors, especially in unflattering light, keep us honest about who we really are: terrific, but also flawed. Every one of us.

This book is intended as the companion volume to *SEEKING THE POSITIVES: A Life Spent on the Cutting Edge of Public Health*, published in late 2015. Whereas that contribution focuses on detailing the exceptional venereal disease (to use the old fashioned label) control accomplishments recorded in Colorado Springs during more than three decades, this slender companion volume focuses on individuals, not strategies. This is a flesh and blood account of some memorable people and some of their experiences while caught up in society's efforts to curtail venereal disease transmission. Although the people featured represent only a tiny proportion of the tens of thousands of people we had the privilege of working with in our control endeavors, the vignettes do provide a graphic sense for the professional world of public health workers toiling in this exciting craft.

First, an apology for using antiquated terminology in this age of "Sexually Transmitted Disease" or, more accurately, "Sexually Transmitted Infection"—for one does not acquire or transmit disease (implying tissue damage), but infection (indicating an infectious agent). Not only does "Venereal Disease" bear a strong relation to this book's title, but the expression is still, after all these years, universally understood. The tried and the true.

What does it take to work in venereal disease control? First, it takes a nonjudgmental energetic person, equipped with a compassionate and empathetic personality, to be successful. Second, it takes courage and persistence. And third, it takes an anthropologist's curiosity.

More than two-dozen people contributed the anecdotes that have been crafted by one of us (JJP) into the 121 vignettes in this collection. Such editing allows for uniformity of style and voice. Each is "signed" using its contributor's initials, except for the few anonymous contributions from, as it were, the "camera shy". Only where essential to understand the vignette's context is the year of the anecdote's occurrence recorded.

Who are these contributors? As suggested by the admittedly scant detail provided in the "List of Contributors" section, virtually all worked as VD/HIV public health workers, either as clinicians or as disease investigators doing contact interviews and actively tracing named partners—for a combined 350 or so years of experience and service.

There is no stereotypic vignette; each is grouped using a shared characteristic into a category: In Clinic, Contact Interviewing, In The Field, HIV/AIDS, Prostitution, and Behind The Scenes. When a vignette can be classified into more than one category, our choice for inclusion is arbitrary. Lots of flavors are offered. Some are funny, some touching, some sad, some tragic, some raunchy (unavoidable, given the subject matter), some revealing, some completely unforgettable, and all (probably) interesting. It's true that some vignettes may be experienced as disturbing or offensive. We worked hard to minimize the impact of some realities—the world has its ugly aspects—and feel that virtually all adult readers can withstand the shock of the (few) disturbing vignettes. Keep in mind that, for better or for worse, there are lots of people in this world who have boundaries that are different from yours. Your reactions will ultimately depend on your personality and, importantly, on which lens you use to focus: the close-up or the long-shot.

Publishing such vignettes—not, to our knowledge, previously done—assumes greater importance when one realizes that the twenty-first century world of sexually transmitted diseases (to use the current nomenclature) control is likelier to be work station- than field-based. Working in an air-conditioned cubicle in an office building using electronic and social media as springboards for control efforts will yield different experiences from those encountered by "shoe-leather" epidemiologists working in situ, in places and neighborhoods where transmission is actually occurring. In brief, this volume's contents may be akin to looking in the rear view mirror rather than through the windshield. The way we were.

Like the goodies in a box of chocolates, this book's vignettes can be savored at random a piece at a time, or several at a time, or (gulp!) in a single sitting—in which case you will neither overdose nor get fat.

Enjoy

John J. Potterat
Nancy E. Spencer
Stephen Q. Muth
September 2017

Acknowledgment

We gratefully acknowledge, and warmly thank, the following people for their contributions to this collection of vignettes:

Anonymous (two people), Devon Brewer, Beth Dillon, Timothy Englert, David Green, Alex Hinst, Rebecca Jordan, Robert Kellner, Patricia Malone, Gary Markewich, Teresa Martinez, Pamela Montoya, Lynanne Plummer, Susan Potterat, Christopher Pratts, Ron Raab, Judith Reynolds, Sandy Rios, Helen Rogers, Shana Hurlbutt Sanderson, Donald Woodhouse, and Helen Zimmerman.

For brief biographical information, see the list of contributors on page 219.

Part I: In Clinic

Commonly referred to as VD (for venereal disease) or STD (for sexually transmitted disease) clinic, it's a specialized public clinic where persons, including minors, can be evaluated for sexually transmitted infection at no, or minimal, cost.

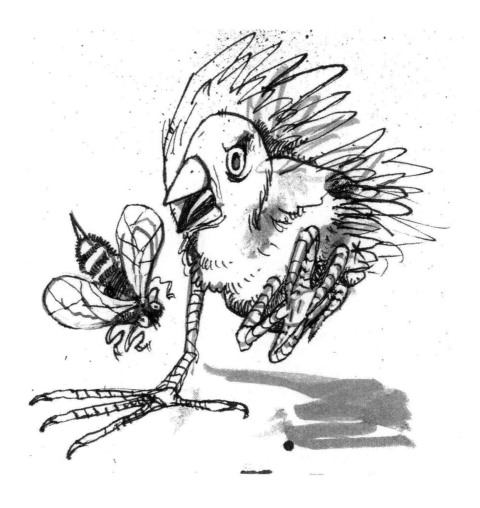

PART I: IN CLINIC

Down There

She's twenty and pretty. Not pretty like Natalie Wood in *West Side Story*, but pretty because youth is pretty. In my presence, she's clearly anxious, uncomfortable. Not because I'm easily twice her age, but because she's sitting across my desk in my VD Clinic in Colorado and (I silently surmise) embarrassed. She comes from Appalachia, where such matters are unlikely to be discussed with men.

A few minutes ago, I welcome her into my office and ask to what pleasure I owe her visit. This is the routine opening line I use with all our patients, for it often serves to quickly relax them. Not Becky. In fact, Becky looks puzzled, as if to ask "What do you mean?" or, perhaps, "Why would this be a pleasure?" I suspect she didn't understand my question; I clarify by asking her why she's here today. Continuing to trace the carpet pattern with her eyes, Becky whispers that she's having problems "down there". Feeling impish, I play her by asking whether it was her feet or knees that were giving her problems. Still disinclined to maintain eye contact, she replies that it's not her legs but, "you know: down THERE". Oh, I reply, you have a stomach ache. Exasperated, she repeats "down THERE" with the same emphatic THERE as before, followed by a few seconds of uncomfortable silence.

I make one more attempt to have Becky accurately locate the source of her medical concern, but have no more luck than before. By now clearly irritated at my (to her, idiotic?) line of questioning, she suddenly raises her head, looks at me dead in the eye, and says: "Down THERE, you know, in my Virginia!"

(JJP)

Why Risk Cutting the Thing You Love Most?

As he swaggers into our VD clinic, Butch looks and acts the part of outlaw motorcycle gang member (which he is): rough, tough, and mean. Moreover, he sports a knife that rivals that of Crocodile Dundee's, probably a foot-and-a-half from top of handle to blade tip. It's tucked inside his right pant leg, with the handle visible above the belt and the blade tip reaching his knee.

I'm a nurse practitioner and he's now sitting in my examination room. I'm clearly uncomfortable in the presence of this intimidating weapon. To avoid stepping on a land mine (as it were) by telling him to remove the knife and place it on the sink a few feet away, I keep my cool and nonchalantly say: "Pull the knife out or you'll cut the thing you love most!" When he sufficiently recovers from the shock of a middle-aged woman saying something like that, I tell him: "Now, let's examine that thing you love most".

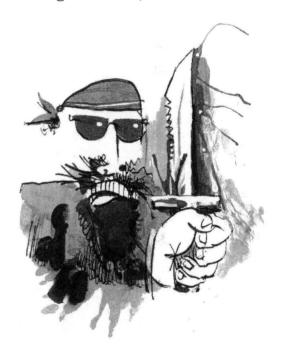

At our clinic meeting, where I relate my encounter, I'm asked about why I state these things so boldly. "Motorcycle gangsters have mothers too" is my reply. It takes a minute or so for staff members to grasp the message: act with maternal authority when you have to.

Lesson in clinic diplomacy learned.

(HPZ)

Middle East Meets Midwest

My daughter is registering patients for our VD clinic in Colorado where I work as a nurse practitioner. It's a part time job for her, an 18-year-old blonde-haired, blue-eyed, pretty college freshman with a ready smile and infectious laugh.

Enter a 30-year-old Arab man visiting from the Middle East, who's instantly smitten when he signs in to register. When his turn comes, I call his name and he acknowledges me by saying: "Here, Sir". Startled, but unfazed, I get basic medical information for this visit (urethral discharge) and send him to be examined and tested for venereal disease.

While he waits for preliminary results from the laboratory, he beckons me, points to the registrar, and asks: "Sir: is she your daughter?" I tell him: "Yes, I'm her mother". "I'll give you two oil wells in my country for your daughter".

Two things puzzle me. How does he find out I'm her parent? I suspect he asks someone in the examination room or laboratory. Above all, why does he address me as "Sir" when I am without a doubt a woman? Too busy to ask, I don't find out the reason for his perception. A bit later I speculate that, because women don't work in his country, he assumes that I must be a man.

Tempting offer? Yes (the money would be nice) but almost exclusively No, since she's my favorite (and only) daughter.

(**HPZ**)

Self-Service Surgery, Warts and All

Carl comes to our VD clinic straight from the county jail where he's been for the last few weeks. When his turn comes, he tells me, the nurse practitioner, that he's "got lots of bumps" on his penis. He's right. On examination, I see that both head and shaft are covered with warts; not only that, but many are surrounded by bloody cuts.

He explains that, while incarcerated, he tries to remove them with a small blade—unsuccessfully at that, but that under no circumstances will he visit the "lousy jail infirmary".

Impatient by nature, Carl is crushed when I tell him that his warts cannot be treated until the cuts, with the help of antibiotics, have healed. It takes more than a week for his messy, self-inflicted surgical wounds to heal and more than a month of weekly treatments for the warts to vanish.

I'm not at all concerned that he might not keep his weekly appointments. His botched self-service surgery, warts and all, teaches him the value of having them correctly treated. His other choice would be to continue self-mutilation, which I privately suspect (read: Masochism? Self-loathing?) has something to do with his initial therapeutic approach.

(HPZ)

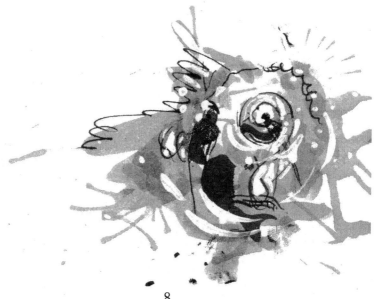

Synagogue Sign Language

I'm a dermatologist moonlighting in the health department's VD clinic; I need the income while I establish my private practice. I'm also Jewish in a medium-sized community with a small Jewish population. There is only one synagogue and getting to know just about everybody is easy.

Right now, I'm entering the room where the nurse has prepared the patient, a teenager, for a pelvic examination: she's flat on her back, eyes on the ceiling, knees raised, ankles in stirrups, a paper sheet covering her pelvic area. I say hello and, as she turns to look at her greeter, she alarmingly utters: "Oh no, not you!" and buries her face in her hands. I chuckle: "You're covering the wrong end". This immediately relaxes her and I spend time reassuring her that I would never talk about this visit to anyone.

Whenever we see each other at synagogue services, we furtively wink. But we never talk about it again, even after all these years.

(GSM)

When Ignorance is a Different Kind of Bliss

Fannie Mae is 16 years old when she comes into our VD clinic and I, the nurse practitioner, ask her what's bothering her. She's worried she might be pregnant because she's very regular and hasn't had a period in 2 months.

The urine sample indicates that this rural Kentucky native is indeed pregnant, a diagnosis that stuns her despite her initial suspicion: "I just couldn't be pregnant; I never let him kiss me".

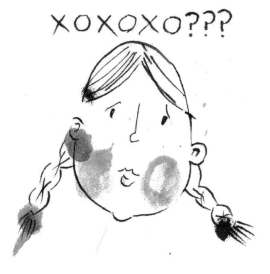

I inform her that pregnancy is exclusively a consequence of unprotected penis-to-vagina sex with ejaculation and that is what happened. Her reply? "Well, my mother told me that if I didn't kiss a guy, I couldn't get pregnant."

So much for her mother's wisdom. This time, it produces a different kind of bliss seven months later: little Jesse.

(HPZ)

Gonorrhea, My Eye!

He's 16 years old and looks and dresses like a street urchin. He's in VD clinic today because of pus copiously draining from one eye. The rapid test indicates gonorrhea infection, which the culture confirms two days later. This diagnosis really surprises him: "Gonorrhea, my eye!"

Ocular gonorrhea is not common. Infection occurs when gonorrhea-contaminated sperm is ejaculated into the face at the moment of climax during oral sex or, sometimes, by gonorrhea-contaminated sperm on fingers that are used to rub an itchy eye.

He insists that he's heterosexual but, to support his heroin addiction, frequently offers men blow-jobs. None of his several (like he, homeless) girlfriends has a positive test for gonorrhea.

And yes, he occasionally gets sprayed in the face during blow-jobs.

(PM)

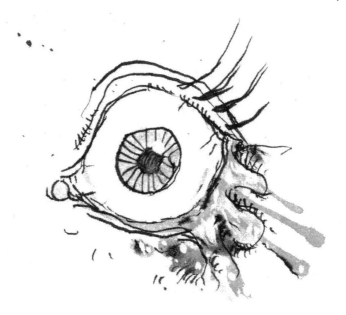

Taming Hard Rider

His hero is Marlon Brando in "The Wild One" and, as he walks into my VD Clinic, he looks the part. He sports a black leather jacket with his motorcycle gang's heraldry emblazoned on the back. He approaches the registrar's desk in a whirlwind wearing his rehearsed, intimidating stare, demanding to be seen right away, because "I'm very busy". Among the dozen fellow patients in the waiting room, squirming is epidemic.

Rude, intrusive behavior does not sit well with our no-nonsense, middle-aged public health nurse. A woman of imposing size in a crisp blue frock, she stands resolutely in front of him, close enough to invade his private space. It's his turn to squirm as she reminds him of the importance of being patient (as I wonder if she is conscious of the play on words) and considerate of others, especially those who are already here. Surprisingly, it's this young hoodlum who is intimidated. He sits and waits his turn. An hour later he leaves, with a barely concealed smile on his tough face, holding a small bottle of pills for his minor infection. End of story? No.

Fast forward two years. This time he has a more serious infection. Because he knows it to be serious, he readily names his contacts and insists on bringing them in personally. And so follows a series of visits by his contacts and his contacts' contacts, including several in his gang, all of whom are mercifully well-behaved in clinic. Grateful for our help in extinguishing this infectious outbreak in his social circles, he personally pledges to kill on my behalf, should such a favor be needed. I make nothing of this memorable remark, simply dismissing it as perhaps typical of motorcycle gang braggadocio.

Many years later, this Brando wannabe and members of his gang are accused by the local police of being hit men for the Mafia. End of story.

(JJP)

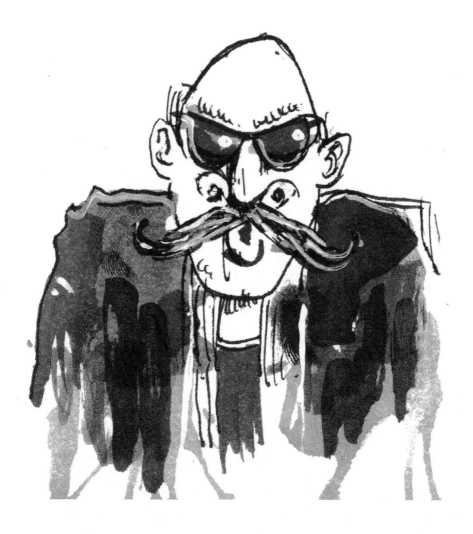

PART I: IN CLINIC

Serious as a Heart Attack

As nurse practitioner in our VD clinic, it's my job to get as accurate a medical history on new patients as possible; Marjorie's should be easy, since she's only 21 years old. Few things go wrong at that age and, certainly, few serious things happen.

Marjorie tells me that she's been out of hospital for two days now. Thinking that this is the reason she's here today, I ask for details. "Heart attack", she replies. Surprised, I ask about family history of cardiovascular disease. "Not that I know of". Because this is the 1980s I unhesitatingly ask: "How long before your heart attack did you use cocaine?" "How did you know?" comes the astonished Marjorie's reaction, but the actual answer is: "A few hours before".

I treat her minor vaginal infection and she goes home.

Is drug abuse serious business? About as serious as a heart attack.

(HPZ)

This Isn't a Lady!

Terrie, aged 32 and freshly arrived from the East Coast, visits our VD clinic for the first time. At high risk by self-report (is she a prostitute?) for venereal infection, Terrie is here for a routine check-up.

Following registration and the minting of a new chart, Terrie is screened by a nurse for standard medical information and then sent to the laboratory for syphilis blood testing (this in pre-AIDS days).

Because Terrie is dressed as a woman, she's assumed to be one and brought into the examination room, directed to sit on the exam table, told to remove her underwear and to position her heels in the stirrups. The attending nurse places a paper sheet over her skirt and tells her to wait for the physician ("She'll be right with you, Terrie").

Enter the physician who greets her, walks over to the business side of the table for the pelvic exam, lifts the sheet and instantly realizes that Terrie has male genitalia. "This isn't a lady" says the physician matter-of-factly to her nurse and refers Terrie to the laboratory for the collection of urethral smear and culture specimens.

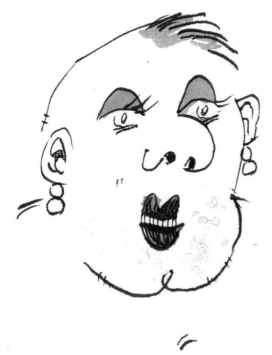

Terrie is amused and laughs loudly, triggering a chain reaction of mirth in the room. "She" is impressed with our staff and returns time and again for regular check-ups. Indeed she now requests to have genital test specimens collected while in the pelvic exam position and, of course, we accommodate her. During the next few years, we learn that cross-dressers (who are becoming more common) may not be anatomically "real" ladies but they're indeed at high risk, as we periodically treat them for syphilis and, especially, gonorrhea.

(HPZ, JR)

Mobile Front Teeth as Occupational Hazard

Stereotyping seems to come naturally to people. I'm no exception. Among patients I casually observe as I stroll through my VD clinic waiting room, for example, there's one kind I classify right away: any young man with mobile front teeth is probably a hockey player. Puck legacy.

When nervously (or impatiently) waiting to be examined, his kind often expresses it by repeatedly pushing the artificial upper front teeth forward and backward, in kitchen drawer fashion, using the tongue.

How reliable is my stereotype? Of the half dozen men I've ever observed with loose front teeth, I've been wrong once (an amateur boxer).

And it doesn't bother me to be proved wrong.

(JJP)

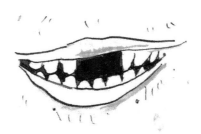

PART I: IN CLINIC

Traditionalist Christian Sect Welcomes New Member

A young man comes into our health department VD clinic with a watery discharge, accompanied with a mild burning sensation, from the tip of his penis. The test confirms chlamydia infection, which puzzles him because his sole sexual partner "cannot possibly have VD" "You see", he continues, "she belongs to a closed traditionalist religious community". He tells me that, weeks ago, he asks to join this "clan" and is accepted by the elders, at which time he donates his worldly possessions, including car, cash, and paychecks. Soon, he makes his interest for a young single woman known to the powers that be, who now approve of the match. Not long after, his genital symptoms appear.

She's treated at a private physician's office without benefit of testing, and I don't get to meet or interview her.

And so the question remains, did she infect this clan's newest member, or did he donate more than his worldly possessions through his own member (as it were), mainly chlamydia?

(PM)

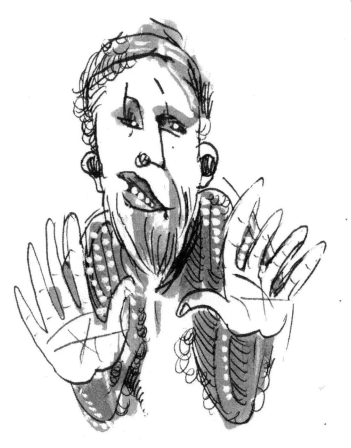

Brothers Who Became Sisters

Corrina, in her mid-twenties, identifies as a woman and presents as a woman. She's born male and retains male genitals. Today I call her, because I'm interested in finding out from whom she recently contracted syphilis and to whom she might have transmitted it. During the phone conversation, she recalls some partners but suggests that I visit her at home, saying that her two roommates should be able to identify more partners, since these three women frequently share different men—not in the three-way, but in the musical chairs, sense. Each is forthcoming about their overlapping partners and responds well to additional probing. Because of partner-sharing I, a woman about their age, recommend that the roommates attend our VD clinic for testing and preventive antibiotic treatment.

Both roommates appear in clinic the next day. It's literally a day of naked reckoning, for my (male) colleague bets that Corrina's roommates are biologically female while I submit that they're probably also born male. Not only does the physical examination confirm my suspicion, but it turns out that one of the roommates is actually Corrina's biological sibling.

Brothers who became sisters!

(NS)

Revolving Door Cherie

I see Cherie for the first time when she comes into our VD clinic complaining of vaginal discharge that won't go away. She's 14 years old, and tells me that she's been sexually active for only few months and that she seldom uses condoms. When I ask her about sexual partners she answers: "Most of the guys are older and give me things so they can have sex with me". Knowing that a young teenager's perception of "older" is likely to differ from mine (I'm nearly forty), she says that although some are in high school, most of them are soldiers at our nearby Army base. A bit later, she tells me that she's confused about her sexuality and that "maybe I'm a lesbian".

As the culture test confirms a few days later, she does have gonorrhea—for the first of many times during the ensuing several years. Future episodes of gonorrhea are also accompanied by concurrent chlamydia, or other genital, infection. These periodic infections occur despite repeated counseling efforts about safer sex by me, as well as by others on our staff.

My frustration is only mildly attenuated by recent research indicating that the adolescent brain processes information differently from that of adults, and that adventurous or/and reckless behavior can be partially accounted for by its pre-adult structure. Maybe it's just ordinary impulsivity or recklessness of youth. What if it has more to do with an emerging psychiatric condition? Is her self-destructive behavior due to brain, mind, or both?

This makes me sad, but mostly concerned about how to successfully counter such revolving door behavior.

(DLG)

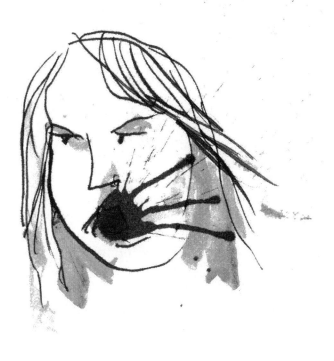

Anatomy Lesson

His wife comes into the emergency clinic, a chunk of flesh in her hand. She hands it to me, a nursing student still in her teens, and asks if I can sew it back on, please. I carry the approximately three-quarters of an inch thick chunk to the physicians' lounge and ask if it can be done. Explosive laughter all around.

It turns out that, in a fit of anger triggered by her husband's chronic philandering, she slices the tip of his penis while he's sleeping off last night's boozing. As we speak, he's anxiously sitting in the waiting room, still bleeding.

Needless to say, the fact that I don't recognize this part of a man's anatomy becomes a source of amusement among the whole staff.

This occurs more than 40 years before the notorious 1993 incident involving John and Lorena Bobbitt. (Nothing new under the sun?)

Anatomy lesson palpably memorized.

PS. The chunk was not sewn back on; reconstructive surgery focused on making a viable urethra.

(HPZ)

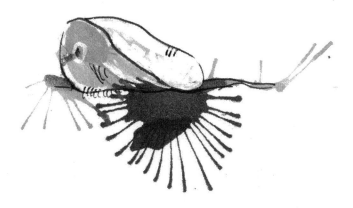

Definitive Definition

He's a precocious, sexually experienced 15-year-old in a detention center waiting his turn to be screened for presence of sexually transmitted diseases by local health department nurses.

Into the private interview room where the boy is waiting enter two nurses: a middle-aged woman on her inaugural training session, here today as a silent observer, and her rapidly-approaching-retirement, seasoned-veteran trainer who does the actual talking.

A brief explanation of procedures is followed by sexual history questions. Of relevance are questions about the ways in which he has sex—vaginally, anally, orally—because this determines the anatomic sites to test. Puzzled by "orally", he asks what she means, and the 65-year-old nurse explains it in polite language, which the boy seemingly fails to understand. Once again, she tries to explain, this time in somewhat less-delicate language. Same result: yet another puzzled look. Exasperated, she rephrases it as: "That's when she sucks your dick or you lick her pussy". His eyes light up. Graphic definition immediately understood.

Instant intergenerational rapport established.

(PZM)

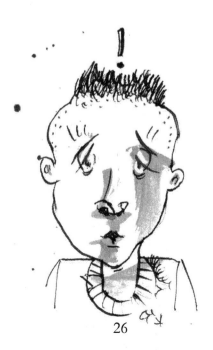

Intersex

I'm in the county jail offering testing for venereal diseases and HIV, as I do periodically on behalf of the local health department. Dana requests testing; I ask the jail nurse where I can find Dana, just as she pulls up a mug shot to familiarize me with my new client: long strawberry-blond hair, freckles, pretty brown eyes, with manicured eyebrows. Dana, a gender-neutral name, is a nice looking woman, in my opinion. Imagine my surprise as she directs me to the male ward.

Dana is a hermaphrodite—now preferably called "intersex". On the outside, he's being privately treated to become the person he really thinks he is, a woman; here, the medical staff refuses to administer his prescribed estrogen injections, because these are not considered medically necessary.

As I meet him, he clearly has secondary syphilis, with textbook-perfect bilateral lesions in his palms, soles of his feet, trunk, and legs. Fortunately, he's soon due for release and able to attend our clinic for syphilis treatment. During the contact interview, he lists both men and women as partners and even claims to have fathered children.

As I fill out the required forms, I realize that I have the same problem the jail authorities have: do I classify Dana as a male or female case for, being behind the times, we do not yet have a category for intersex.

(Anonymous)

PART I: IN CLINIC

IN THE SHADOW OF VENUS

Part II: Contact Interviewing

Identifying the sexual partners of patients with VD/STD is important, because this allows public health workers to find out where the infection came from (looking upstream) and where it may have been forwarded (downstream). This process is completely confidential.

IN THE SHADOW OF VENUS

PART II: CONTACT INTERVIEWING

How Much Time Do I Gotta Serve for This?

He's an attractive, kind, concerned man in his thirties, recently diagnosed with syphilis in its early, most-infectious stage. Among my other duties as his case manager, I'm charged with assuring that his sexual partners are confidentially informed of possible exposure to this serious, yet easily curable, disease. I explain that we need to find out not only from whom he acquired infection (what patients usually focus on), but also to whom it may subsequently have been transmitted (what patients reluctantly, if at all, ever think about). Unlike most syphilis patients, he readily understands this need and cooperates with minimal prompting by me.

A short while later, he suddenly folds his hands together, places his elbows on his knees, looks straight at me and asks: "How much time do I gotta serve for this?" Startled, a few seconds elapse before I realize he's thinking that transmitting syphilis to others is a criminal offense, punishable by incarceration! My heart fills with empathy and, yes, even sadness. I also realize that his question represents an opportunity and that I could respond with: "Well, that depends on how many sexual partners you tell me about!" Being neither a cynic nor an opportunist, I instead explain that this sort of punishment might have been meted out centuries ago but that today, syphilis is simply a manageable public health problem. Visibly relieved, he continues listing his sexual partners.

(NS)

Magnetic

She must send "Come on" signals everywhere she goes, even at work. A not unattractive teenager, her threshold for acceptance is nevertheless low. In a recent three-month period, she tells me that she reclines with about a dozen young men—the likely reason she winds up in our VD clinic. But I'm getting ahead of myself.

Of infected people, chlamydia is most frequently diagnosed in adolescent women. Camellia is such a patient, and I'm presently interviewing her for sexual partner information. I recruit her for a study of enhanced interviewing techniques aimed at helping patients remember *all* of their sexual partners. In the standard part of the interview, she names only two partners, but after I start using a series of experimental memory-prompting cues, she recalls nearly a dozen more.

Amazed at the effectiveness of different interviewing cues to jog her memory, Camellia excitedly exclaims: "OK, this is a good game!", "Oh my God! I can't believe all this stuff is coming back now!", and "This is really working!" She unabashedly details specific length-of-sexual-exposure features: "Two strokes, that's it!"; "I was humping all day"; "With him? Maybe three strokes"; "He was fine, but he stunk"; or "It was gross".

This impulsive adolescent met these men in diverse places: police checkpoints ("he was the policeman"), night clubs ("he works in the back"), restaurants ("he was my server"), among other, diverse, settings. After mentioning only half of the partners she ultimately recalls, she glances at my notes and gasps: "Oh my gosh, the list is that long?"

In some instances she can't remember their first names and, in a few cases, she doesn't even *know* their first names.

(PZM, DDB)

Running the Womens

He's in the Army, after having lived most of his 22 years in an eastern seaboard inner city. Today, he shows up in my dispensary with a discharge. Not the honorable, military kind, but the painful urethral kind. While waiting for the rapid smear result, I ask if he's ever had something like that before. "No, not VD, but something called Non-Specific Uterus." I know now that he's not a stereotypical patient and look forward to finding out more about his life, especially his sex life, since the smear comes back positive. It's gonorrhea and, hence, I need to determine from whom he got the infection and to whom he may have passed it on.

He says he doesn't know, because he's had lots of partners. Fascinated, I ask him what makes him so successful at bedding so many. He says that women like to talk and that he accommodates them. For what I suspect is emphasis, he tells me that "I always conversate them before I sex them". By now I'm in heaven; this soldier is refreshingly original. He's making my day. After obtaining locating information on his partners, I ask him about his plans after discharge. He tells me he has a 5-year-old son living with his mother and that, in a couple of years, he'll be ready to father him. Curious, I ask him what he means, to which he replies: "I'm gonna teach him how to run the womens."

(DEW)

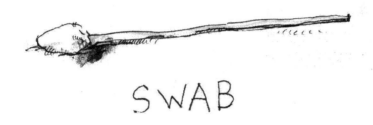

The Beauty and the Beast

She's an attractive teenager who's in our VD clinic because one of her sexual partners has syphilis. Two days later, the test results show that she has three infections: syphilis, gonorrhea, and chlamydia, a rare "hat trick", as it were.

Thinking that none of her three recent sexual partners can possibly have a dreadful disease like syphilis, she tells me, the health department interviewer, that her "dog may have given me syphilis, because my dog gives me oral sex".

Sniffilis?

(**SQM**, **Anonymous**)

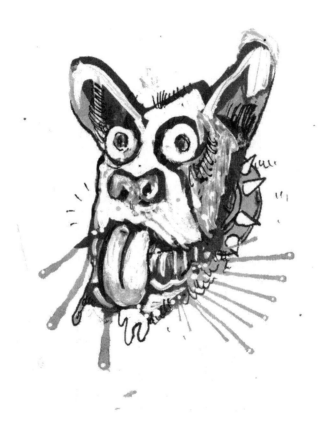

The Fourth Man

What takes me by surprise is that she nonchalantly lists him as the fourth of five sexual partners for the last six months. Seemingly nobody special. Carla has

PART II: CONTACT INTERVIEWING

syphilis and (at this point) she's being asked to provide only the first name of each sexual partner. Last names and locating information are customarily solicited last, to discourage patients from the temptation of withholding names of "important" people.

Four of the five partners are, like her, ordinary young people of college age. The fourth man's last name suggests that of a popular musician, which Carla confirms when asked about his occupation. She doesn't know his address, but volunteers to point out his house, which is not far from our VD clinic. To avoid the frustration of driving in this neighborhood's labyrinthine streets, I ask for a phone number. For the first time in the interview, Carla seems reluctant to cooperate. Pressed, she reveals that the phone number is a direct line to his bedroom and that he'll therefore "know who gave him syphilis". I reassure her that she's neither likely to be the only sexual partner with that phone number nor, probabilistically, to have infected him. Relieved, she gives me the phone number.

I call him the next day just before noon; he answers, wanting to know how I got his number. I explain that we at the health department are not allowed to reveal this information and that the important thing is for him to know that he's involved in a syphilis outbreak and needs a blood test to protect his health. Surprisingly, given his prominence, he readily cooperates and, additionally, is fun to talk with.

To his relief, he tests negative.

(**JJP**)

Holly Roller

I know this syphilis patient is going to be challenging, for I've yet to meet a minister with venereal disease who is voluble about its origin. Experience tells me that a man of the cloth with VD is behaviorally as flawed as the rest of us. The challenge is to get him to tell me, the health department VD contact tracer, the truth and nothing but the truth. Great expectation!

Delbert is forty, pudgy, and pasty complexioned. He cagily ducks my trying to meet him, preferring to discuss his case by phone. I insist on meeting him in person, the better to read his defenses. He reluctantly consents, and we meet in an out-of-town restaurant, in a secluded booth. He's wearing a white suit, his trademark attire as a charismatic fundamentalist preacher. He looks creepy and, as a young woman, I feel uncomfortable at the way he inspects me. In whispers, he denies any sexual exposures. This is when I suggest that his reason for denial is that he's having sex with men—the most common sexual profile of men with syphilis in our city. He does not deny it but simply stays silent every time I mention it (often). Exasperated at my persistence, he finally confesses to having had sex with three teen-aged girls in his congregation during the period of interest (the last 6 months).

The telephone numbers he provides are genuine and each girl consents to examination. Each independently volunteers that Delbert must be the infected person. Not being in the confirmation business, I focus on directing them to a blood testing facility. None of the three teens is positive for syphilis. I suspect that Delbert is having sex with anonymous male partners, which is why he sees no point in admitting it. Yet another unproductive, frustrating case.

That evening, while watching "Elmer Gantry", the film adaptation of Nobel Prize winner Sinclair Lewis's 1927 novel about an unscrupulous minister inclined to sexual predation, I think about how "rolling Hollies" by charismatic ministers is certainly not new. Nor, do I suspect, is it likely to stop. Holly Roller, indeed.

(BAD)

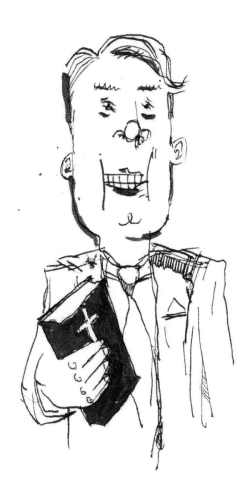

Much Better the Second Time Around

She's 83, a real lady, and lives like one. She's being diagnosed with early syphilis at her private doctor's office, where the plan is to cure her infection with two shots of penicillin in her buttocks, a blessing of modern medicine.

My colleague and I, both women in our twenties working for the health department, are presently in her well-appointed house to interview her for sexual partner information. She's visibly upset, mostly angry at herself at what she construes as bad judgment—dating an attractive man about twenty-five years her junior, whom she met in church a few months ago.

Handkerchief in hand, tears in her eyes, nose dripping lightly, she says that this is the second time she's being diagnosed with early syphilis. The first occurred 60 years ago when the only treatment was a year-long regimen of weekly "hip and arm" shots consisting of heavy metals (bismuth, mercury) and arsenic, a metalloid. ("I can still, after all these years, remember the metallic taste of these treatments.") She describes the pain of these shots and, crucially, the humiliation of standing in a long line on the street outside the general hospital clinic, where everybody knew why you were in that specific queue.

Every cloud has a silver lining: there are indeed some things related to Venus that are much better the second time around.

(BAD, NS)

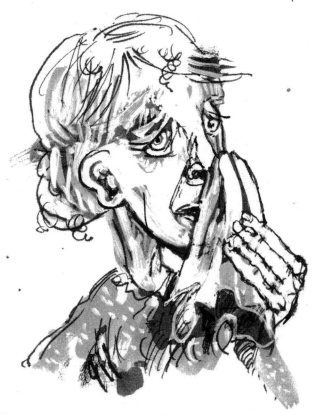

PART II: CONTACT INTERVIEWING

Rare Beast: Teen AIDS

Jermaine is a 17-year-old high school student with HIV. Such an infection is rarely seen in teens[1], and I'm puzzled, as well as curious, about its origin. Our HIV control program is conscientiously tracking all reported cases, and our data reliably show that the typical male patient with HIV acquires it about 10 years later, at age 27 or 28.

He's tested at a local hospital when he complains of pain and not feeling well. Because he's a recent arrival to our high altitude (6,300 feet) city from rural Mississippi, he's given a series of tests, including one for sickle cell anemia. Only the HIV test is positive.

To discuss his infection, risk factors, and at-risk partners, I meet him in a private office at school rather than at home or my health department office. He admits to a few typical teen sexual encounters with, by definition, other low-risk teens—but none

---

[1] Increasing mean age of HIV cases argues against increased transmission or susceptibility among young people. Potterat JJ, Woodhouse DE, Rothenberg RB, Muth SQ, Darrow WW, Muth JB, Reynolds JU. AIDS in Colorado Springs: is there an epidemic? *AIDS* 1993; 7: 1517–1521 (Table 2 & p. 1520, top).

involving high-risk exposures: sex with other men or/and injecting drug use. He adamantly denies such exposures and only after persistent questioning and cajoling does he tell me about homosexual encounters—all with older family members who forced him into sex beginning in childhood. Predictably he's told never to reveal such encounters to anyone... or else.

Now I know why he leaves his Mississippi family to live here, with safer relatives.

(DLG)

Top to Bottom

He's masculine and a box-office draw. He's presently being named as a sexual partner by a teenaged hustler, Damien, whom we're currently treating for syphilis at our health department's VD clinic. During the interview, Damien tells me that this actor appears regularly at a popular gay venue where Damien sells his sexual services. He reveals that he and fellow hustlers find it ironic that this top man is preferentially bottom man in their sexual encounters. Whatever the distance between the ideal and the real, Damien says the money the actor offers is "really good".

When I contact the actor the next day, he agrees to get checked at his private doctor's office, where he's shown to be negative for syphilis, from top to bottom.

(JJP)

An Investigatory Shot in the Dark

Taylor is being diagnosed with first-stage syphilis in our VD clinic. He's now sitting in my interview room, a young homosexual who (predictably, for it happens so often) claims only anonymous partners in a local gay bathhouse. Although he professes not to know anything about the men he has sex with, I ask for his forbearance while I ask some questions about them. I tell him that what is marginal information to you is working information for me.

Taylor's last sexual exposure being three weeks ago and, because this specific partner fits perfectly as likely source for his fresh infection, I focus intently on obtaining potentially-useable locating information. I ask lots of questions, including silly ones, like whether zodiacal-sign information was exchanged. It eventually comes out that the partner lives in Steubenville and that he works in a restaurant that does not serve breakfast, on Belvedere Boulevard. This critical piece of information is revealed when Taylor suggests accompanying him to work (for it is now early morning at the bathhouse) and sharing breakfast with him.

Without even the contact's first name, I nevertheless scribble a personal note about needing to talk with him about a serious health matter, stuff it in a blank envelope, and start cruising up and down Belvedere Boulevard looking for a restaurant that does not serve breakfast. I finally see a deli I surmise does not do breakfast, enter and notice a young man behind the counter. This may well be the guy, so I ask him if he's from Steubenville. "Yes I am". Bingo! I hand him the unaddressed envelope, telling him to read it later. When he calls, he uses his first name to ask for me. One part of the name down, one to go. After explaining that he's a contact to a syphilis patient, I ask him to spell his last name so I can register him in clinic in advance. And he does: S-M-I-T-H. I apologize for asking, lamely explaining that some spell the name S-M-Y-T-H.

This shot in the dark yields another dividend: his test does come back positive for syphilis.

(BAD)

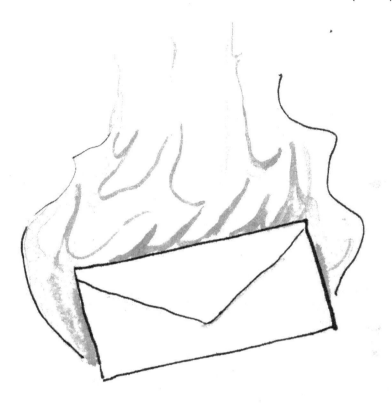

Likely Story

This morning I receive a report from our local U.S. Air Force base requesting help in locating the civilian sexual partner of an airman recently diagnosed with gonorrhea. Darnell tells the military nurse that he probably "picked it up from a prostitute not far from a downtown 7-11 store". Likely story, for it often serves as a cover to conceal homosexual exposure—at the time forbidden fruit in the military. I call the nurse to ask for permission to interview Darnell in person. Granted. A few hours later, he and I meet in a private room on base, where I assure him that sexual partner information is not shared with the military, especially if sexual partners are other men, as I (tell him I) suspect. He's adamant that he's not fabricating a story, and insists on driving to the downtown location to point out where she lives. After a few false stops while driving for half an hour in what he claims to be her neighborhood—which raises my suspicion that this is an elaborate ruse—he finally points to the third floor alley apartment where they had sex.

Armed with a detailed description of the nameless prostitute, I knock firmly on the apartment door.

When a woman fitting Darnell's description answers the door, I (also a young woman) ask her to come into the hall where I can speak to her in private, out of earshot from the man sitting on her couch. She agrees without hesitation. I tell her that I'm not absolutely sure I'm speaking to the right person but urge her to come to the clinic for venereal disease testing, because I suspect she's been exposed. Again, she agrees without hesitation.

Both she and her man-friend attend the clinic that afternoon, where she's diagnosed as having a pelvic infection, which proves to be gonorrhea. As is customary, her man-friend is simultaneously treated.

A likely story is sometimes just that.

(BAD)

We Don't Snitch

Many people reside in the United States illegally. For understandable reasons, being approached by a government agency such as ours, the health department, is a source of anxiety and defensiveness when such persons are named as at-risk partners to STD or HIV patients. Experience from their country of origin teaches them to be wary of any government agency, even if it's one ethically and legally bound by medical confidentiality as we routinely, and in plain language, aim to reassure them: "You can trust us; we don't snitch".

I'm in the backroom of a minority neighborhood bar with Rita who, like me, is a woman in her late twenties. She has pelvic inflammatory disease, a fertility-threatening consequence of gonorrhea bacteria reaching the Fallopian tubes from the cervix. As I interview her for partner information, I begin to suspect that her boyfriend is both infected (but without visible genital symptoms) and, perhaps, an illegal alien. The interview is almost finished when she agitatedly warns me: "You need to leave. I don't know how else to say this, but you need to leave NOW!" I see no sign of danger but nevertheless ask if she is in trouble and needs help. After she says "No" it takes but a split second for me to realize that it is I who is the trouble. Her boyfriend is unexpectedly entering the bar and she knows very well that he doesn't want Rita to talk to "The Man".

We complete our conversation the next day by telephone. I emphatically urge her to make sure her boyfriend is treated, if only to avoid re-infection and the attendant risk of infertility.

Deep-seated distrust is not infrequently encountered by infectious disease contact tracers in areas well-represented by illegal residents, even after assurances are proffered that "We don't snitch".

(NS)

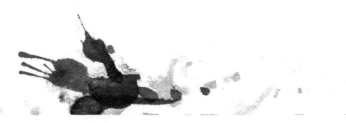

Goody Two-Shoes

Madison is seemingly the ideal teen: strikingly beautiful, blonde-haired, blue-eyed, vivacious, and professing the virtuous life. She may well be the envy of all blue-blooded American parents. That's the "A" side of the record.

I'm more familiar with the "B" side. I work for the VD control program at the local health department. Madison is being named as a sexual partner of a young inner-city gang member being diagnosed with VD as we speak. We know Madison must be infected, because two other infected gang members also name her this week. Each mentions her exceptional enthusiasm as a giver of oral sex, admittedly an inefficient means of transmitting VD. Nevertheless, we need to locate her since inefficient does not mean impossible; regrettably none of the 3 young men claims to know where she lives or how to reach her.

Two weeks later, a student at a military academy is diagnosed at the cadet clinic with the same genital infection, naming Madison as his only sexual partner, specifying the "sex" as only fellatio. He relates that she fellated him last Sunday at the church picnic after the religious service, in her car's back seat in the church parking lot. Fortunately he knows exactly how to locate her, because she lives in the same upper middle class neighborhood and attends the same church.

"Goody Two-Shoes" refers to a person, usually a girl, who's conservative in dress and behavior, takes pride in her virginity, practices abstinence (generally referring to sex occurring below her waist, front or back), is God-fearing, and goes to church every Sunday.

Yes, that's indeed Madison's "A" side.

Side "B" we treat at the clinic with antibiotics and advice about safer behaviors.

(SQM)

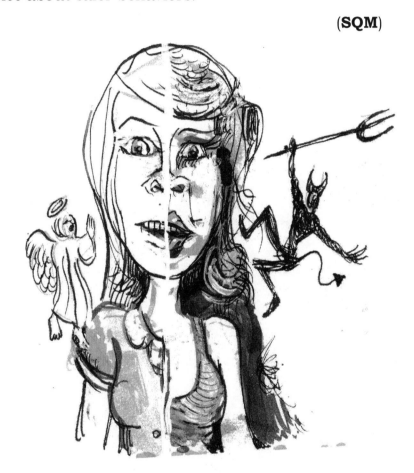

Whoever Heard of Gonorrhea of the Elbow?

If it happens, you can bet it occurs late on a Friday afternoon, just before Happy Hour at workweek's end. It's usually an urgent or unusual case reported telephonically to my department, venereal disease control, by a local hospital. On this Friday afternoon, my supervisor sends me to interview a young woman hospitalized because of disseminated gonorrhea, an uncommon complication of this disease.

The moment I introduce myself in her hospital room, she blurts out: "Whoever heard of gonorrhea of the elbow? I don't have sex with my elbows!" Being both young women with a good sense of humor, we laugh at this preposterous idea. Very relaxing.

I explain that gonorrhea occasionally makes its way from genital organs into the blood stream, setting up housekeeping in the synovial fluid in joints like knees and elbows. Although I'm tempted to ask her with whom she's been rubbing elbows, I concentrate on having her identify sexual partners, since some are likely to be infected without obvious symptoms.

And yes, I make it in time to rub elbows as customary with my coworkers at a local bar for Friday happy hour.

(NS)

PART II: CONTACT INTERVIEWING

Every Tom, Dick, and Harry

George, nearly 60 years old, is one of the first volunteers for our study on how injection drug users recall the people they shoot drugs with. He's referred to our study from another public health study on injection drug use. His decades of injecting drugs and cerebral, candid manner make me think of him as the wise godfather of the local scene.

When I ask him to estimate the number of people with whom he's injected drugs during the last 2 years, George answers: "about a thousand" and explains that "I know everybody in this fucking town and all of the dope addicts". When I ask him to list as many injection partners as he can by name, he balks: "I can't answer this question. I refuse to tackle it, it's just too big... it's not the point that I don't want to identify 'em or tell the right straight thing about it, but like you can just start writing first names down and that would cover (it)... naming Charlie and Joe and Tom and Dick and Harry, this, this would be the whole situation right here".

George describes how he typically injects with others he knows only by face and previous interactions, and that even street names are not exchanged. After I further encourage him, he eventually lists 22 by first name.

Near the end of the interview he schools me by revealing his secrets to success as a drug addict: always inject safely (in ways that prevent exposure to others' blood); interact anonymously with other addicts (so they can't identify you to police or someone with ill intent); never commit a crime to support drug use (because drug use is not possible in jail); share your drugs (so others will share when you have none); and simply keep yourself together when you cannot get drugs (live to use drugs; don't use drugs to live).

Despite a long history of injection with innumerable partners, I suspect he survives as well as he does precisely because he's lived by these principles.

(DDB)

PART II: CONTACT INTERVIEWING

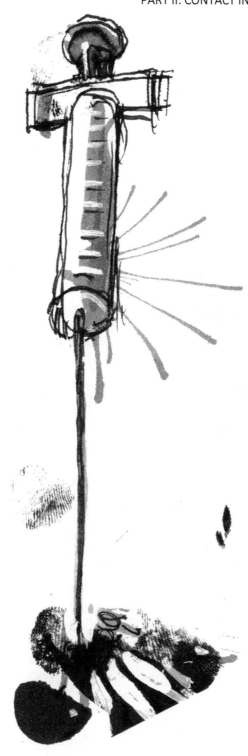

IN THE SHADOW OF VENUS

Part III: In the Field

Tracing the sexual partners of patients with venereal disease often takes the public health worker out of the office and into "the field". The idea is to locate exposed persons where they live or socialize. Discretion and confidentiality are the procedure's bedrock.

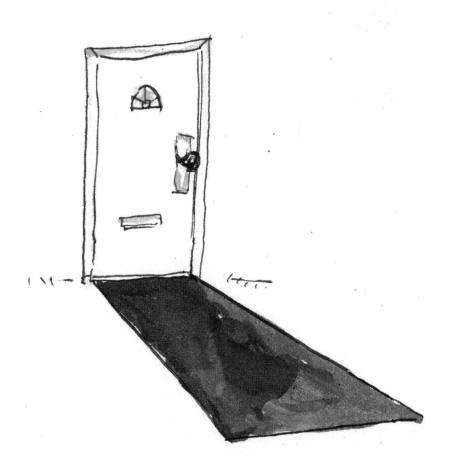

PART III: IN THE FIELD

Gonorrhea Transmission Live (Almost!)

Health department sleuths (like me) who trace the sexual partners of people with VD are usually weeks, if not months, downstream from the actual transmission events. It never crosses my mind that I might ever witness such an event live.

I arrive at Consuela's house midmorning on a depressingly overcast day. I'm here to inform her that the routine screening test done a few days ago is positive for gonorrhea. I ring the bell. The door opens and an older woman, who I presume to be her mother, tells me that Consuela is in the upstairs bedroom on the left. (Were I not a young woman, I doubt "mother" would have invited me in.)

The bedroom door is ajar. I notice a fully-clothed young couple, one of whom is Consuela, cuddling on the bed. For privacy, I motion her to meet me in the hallway; once told she has gonorrhea, she agrees to have me drive her to the VD clinic to be treated. She puts her coat on and starts for the stairs. It was just then I say, as I presume the young man is also her lover: "We need to bring him also!" And we do.

This is the only time in my 25-year VD career that I (almost) got to see gonorrhea in the making.

(**NS**)

La Diabla Aquí

I'm a contact tracer in VD clinic, and my job is to notify people who are exposed to sexually transmitted disease. I'm a very tall, fortyish, slender woman of Irish ancestry. I also am fluent in Spanish. For a few weeks, I tenaciously try to reach a young pregnant (hence my persistence) Latina named Maria who's been exposed to chlamydia, an infection which can lead to spontaneous abortion or damage the baby at birth. Several phone messages to Maria, followed by several confidential notes I leave at her apartment at different times, fail to get a response.

Not easily discouraged, I make yet another visit to Maria's residence and, this time, someone opens the door. She is an older Latina woman who, when I ask her if Maria is home, rolls her eyes and yells: "Maria, la diabla aquí" ("Maria, the she-devil is here").

Unfazed, I ask her, in fluid Spanish, how she's feeling, while thanking her for her help in summoning Maria. She rapidly leaves the room, taking her embarrassed face with her, as Maria makes an appreciated appearance.

(**PZM**)

Unusual Night Train

It's January 1983, and Denver is not only experiencing one of its coldest snaps on record, but also an outbreak of syphilis among older, heterosexual street alcoholics. This is unusual, because local syphilis cases are typically diagnosed in young gay men. There are two strikes against health department sleuths (us) being able to successfully find sexual partners: being alcohol impaired makes it difficult for infected persons to recall or clearly identify partners, while being mostly homeless makes it difficult to locate them even if accurately named.

We use the unusual strategy of assuming that possible sex partners, friends and other associates of diagnosed syphilis cases in this small, local subculture are at high risk of infection and should be invited for blood testing. Two of us, each in our early thirties and each of the opposite sex, hit the brutally cold (usually way below zero) streets, attempting to find people connected to that group, each of whom, in turn, is given the opportunity to point out others who might be connected and could benefit from being tested.

The Strange Attractor during this month of freezing temperatures is, understandably, a neighborhood liquor store, which opens at the unusual hour of 8am. And so, several days a week, the two of us appear at opening time. Because we are told that the beverage of choice in this group is *Night Train*, we pay particular attention to people who buy this beverage and who fit the description of people we are looking for. Each day we escort those who volunteer to be tested to our nearby VD clinic, where we also ask them to name others who might be involved. When done, we often drive each volunteer to the local soup kitchen. One day, while visiting a bar frequented by some members of this group, we draw bloods in the privacy of its bathroom, with some patients actually drawing their own blood, a skill acquired because they're injecting drug users and therefore know the location of accessible veins. The one who breaks our hearts is Crystal, who lives in a dumpster and is easily recognized by the disfiguring injury inflicted in childhood by her mother.

It takes a full month of shoe-leather contact tracing in brutally cold weather before we run out of persons to test and declare the outbreak over. In a self-congratulatory mood, we buy a bottle of *Night Train*, brown-bag it, and drink it in our office as we cope with the substantial paperwork documentation.

We thus dare disturb two universes: that of street alcoholics and that of office protocols against alcohol use on the premises. This proves an unusual instance of win-win daring.

(NS, BAD)

In the Swing

It's Friday evening at the VD clinic, and he's now being informed of his syphilis diagnosis. A ruggedly handsome, single, white heterosexual man in his early forties, he's clearly shaken by this unwelcome, if not unexpected, news. He's also a swinger, which he reveals during the contact interview when unable to identify his sexual partners. Genuinely concerned about the implications of the diagnosis for the health of others, he asks for advice about what can be done to notify his anonymous partners. As a first step it's suggested that he call fellow swingers who are his buddies to see if they might know his partners' identities. Two calls are presently made, with the predictable reaction of shock and disbelief at the receiving end, but followed with a promise to be tested and to help notify others in the club even in the absence of knowing their names. Because sexual partner anonymity is the major impediment to controlling this outbreak, it's the right time for the trial balloon: would he facilitate our being invited to screen club members for syphilis via blood testing? He readily agrees to be the go-between and soon obtains permission from the club's owner for health department infectious disease staff to offer testing on the busiest night (Saturday) of the coming weekend.

Our staff consists of two young women and a slightly older man. In the early evening, we arrive at the current week's location for this swingers' club rendezvous. It's a ranch house in Denver's suburbs, where the lighting is low and each bedroom has a double bed with fresh linen. The owner invites us to set up shop in the (well-lit) kitchen area, telling us to feel at home. Everyone agreeing to be tested is friendly, showing up dressed with only a towel. Feeling uncomfortable and out of sorts because we are fully clothed I, the youngest woman, break the ice and announce that I'm taking my clothes off and donning a towel! The other two staff members immediately follow suit (pun intended).

Being on the same sartorial footing as the people we invite, we deal with the now brisk demand, blood-testing swingers until past midnight.

(**NS**, **RK**)

You're Too Dumb to Charge

One of the appealing things about VD contact tracing is the opportunity it provides to meet people you're unlikely to meet any other way.

LaDonna is one of them. She calls me at home on Saturday afternoon wanting to know about the note slipped under her apartment door yesterday. Who am I and what do I want? I explain that I work for the health department and am contacting her about her probable exposure to gonorrhea. After the stereotypic questions ("I have what?", "How do you know?", "Who gave you my name?") LaDonna assures me that "I don't have no gungarita". I explain that, because their reproductive organs are inside, and because the cervix has no pain centers, women can easily have VD without obvious symptoms. This explanation fails to register, as she continues to insist that: "I know my body, I know my pussy, and I ain't got nothin' ".

Because sometimes the best defense is offense, she redirects the conversation by telling me: "You work for the health department? I bet you give your pussy away for free!", breaking out into a belly laugh loud enough that my boyfriend, half a room away, can easily hear. She continues taunting me: "You're too dumb to charge. You gotta be smart not to give your pussy away for free. Hah hah hah hah hah!"

The idea that a woman has sex and doesn't charge is, to LaDonna, hilarious, not to mention beyond absurd. I can still hear her laughing so hard that I'm willing to bet she has tears in her eyes and (probably) even wets herself.

Fortunately, reason prevails as LaDonna shows up in VD clinic on Monday, where she's treated for exposure to gonorrhea pending the test result two days later. And yes, her culture is positive for gonorrhea.

(RJ)

Awakening

What's a nice girl like me doing applying for a job like this? Tracing the partners of sexually transmitted disease (STD) cases, mostly in the field, sounds rewarding. For openers, being a suburban, single mom with three school-aged kids, I desperately need full-time work; for another, the idea of working with people and not being stuck in an office all day fits my preferences.

Basic training takes a breathtakingly short two weeks. It consists of intensive lectures on STD, of motivational interview techniques, of phlebotomy (drawing blood), and being drilled on the importance of rapid response ("Peppy Epi"—contacting named partners within three days).

It's my first time out in the field, and the person I'm looking for lives in a poor, crime-ridden part of Denver (where I grew up) that I have never dared drive through, even with windows rolled up and doors locked. I cannot believe that, arriving at the address, I'm actually getting out of my car, alone, and walking up the steps to the stranger's front door. It's late afternoon. My knees are shaking. I ring the doorbell. To my great relief: no answer! I scribble a personal note, slip it under the door and, as I rush for the safety of my car, I notice the smell of chicken frying somewhere and I hear kids laughing as they play a short distance from me. I suddenly realize that the sun is still shining and that the street is peaceful. It occurs to me that people in this neighborhood may not be very different from me.

This initial field visit changes me forever.

(AH)

Cry the Beloved Mother

A young man arrested for pimping in Colorado, he's jailed and, as part of in-processing, screened for gonorrhea. By the time his test comes back positive, he's no longer there; it's my job to find him for treatment. Because the phone number he provides is disconnected, I drive to the address listed in the reverse directory for that number. I, a young white woman, ring the bell; the door is answered by two black women, one considerably older than the other. The younger woman (his sister, it turns out) says that he no longer lives here but, concerned that there might be something wrong, invites me into the house. Bound by confidentiality, I tell them non-specifically that I need to reach him about a health matter. At least they now are relieved to know that this is not a criminal matter. Yet, no sooner said, the older woman (his mother, it turns out) looks at me sorrowfully, taking her handkerchief out of her dress pocket, and slumps onto the couch, sobbing softly. Because AIDS has been in the news a lot lately, she must be assuming the worst. I reassure both women that this is not about a very serious health matter and that he will be OK once I reach him. The sister presently leaves the room and quickly returns with a crumpled piece of paper with his current address in California (yet another county jail, it turns out). Both seem relieved and happy that I'll help make things right.

As I turn to bid them goodbye, I feel goose bumps with the warm thought that even pimps' mothers cry for their sons.

(NS)

Unto the Next Generation?

As a nurse practitioner and contact tracer for the health department's sexually transmitted diseases program, I meet people both as patients in the clinic and as contacts "in the field".

I'm in the field now, looking for a 16-year-old girl recently named as a sexual partner to a young man with chlamydia. I drive up to the house where she lives and knock on the door, which is answered by a woman in her late thirties who unhesitatingly says: "Doreen, which one of my kids do you need to see?" Startled, but cognizant of my duty to medical confidentiality (Colorado law protects minors in matters of venereal exposure) I reply: "The fact that I'm here doesn't mean there's a problem. I'm just checking to make sure Tanya is O.K." The mother smiles at my explanation and asks about the next clinic session.

She brings both of her daughters to the clinic the next day and couldn't be nicer, either to the staff she's met before about twenty years ago, or to her daughters.

I've worked here longer than I'm inclined to admit when I begin to take care of the next generation's exposures to venereal infection, as do many of my long-term colleagues, STD Lifers like me!

(HPZ)

Why Did You Wait So Long?

There are days in my professional life as a sexually transmitted diseases tracker that I feel burned out, usually from the dispiriting task of tracking down infected people who provide phony locating information—not to mention other lies—to me and our VD clinic staff.

This week is a doozy. I start burning out early on Wednesday and my batteries aren't recharged until Friday, by which time I need to kick ass and make up for two days of shoddy productivity. My first call is to a young woman (like me) who has a positive gonorrhea test, whom I should have notified as soon as the test result was known two days ago, when I was feeling miserable. Once told, she asks me why the delay informing her. Although I reply (truthfully) that I don't always receive results from the laboratory promptly, I don't have the courage to tell her that this failure was (inexcusably) my fault. Shame on me.

Hard lesson well learned, for I never ever let that happen again.

(NS)

Double (Triple?) Jeopardy

Did you fall out of your tree?

This is my unbelieving reaction when Gary approaches me, his supervisor in the VD Program, with a no-brainer question. I immediately read the low energy and disinterest in his indifferent gaze. He explains that a young man—just named as the sole sexual partner of a woman with a serious infection (gonorrhea in the Fallopian tubes)—is the same person named about a month prior in an identical case, at which time he refuses Gary's offer to be examined or treated. Gary presently seeks my permission to administratively close the paperwork as "refused examination", based on last month's encounter; his fallacious reasoning is that "once uncooperative, always uncooperative".

My unbelief turns to disappointment, as I silently blame myself for poor professional mentoring. I recover quickly from pointing the finger at myself to redirecting it where it properly belongs as I frustratingly blurt out: "This guy transmitted serious infection to two women of childbearing age, and you want to turn tail? Go out and get him NOW and bring his ass into the clinic, so that we can prevent him from infecting a third."

A properly-raised young woman, I'm surprised at my intemperate choice of words, but it gets the job done.

(NS)

Quality Control

Medicine is a virtue-based profession. A physician diagnoses and treats a condition and I, as infectious disease investigator, act as physician extender by addressing a diagnosis' public health implications. Hence, venereal disease contact tracing (my job) is also virtue-based and subject to standard medical ethics.

Each profession has members who fall short of expectations. Lenny is one of them. He's a well-trained and experienced VD contact tracer who, after about a year on the job, shows worrisome evidence of low quality work. Things apparently improve as several coworkers, including me, coach and encourage him to do better.

Trusting is fine, but verifying is better. Therefore, I'm asked by our supervisor to verify entries that Lenny logs for his field assignments. The first person I contact has gonorrhea, but tells me that no one has let her know, contradicting Lenny's dated entry on the required (for medico-legal reasons) paperwork. Wanting to believe Lenny, I rationalize this incident by telling myself that it's probably a fluke. I move on to several other "completed" and "properly documented" work assignments. The second, third, fourth, and fifth persons contacted each tell a similar story: no one's informed them of their exposure or need to be treated for venereal disease. Lenny "explains" each instance, but I soon realize that the only consistency in his excuses is inconsistency. He lies. And lies. And then lies some more.

Loaded with desirable attributes for his job—college degree (did he cheat his way through?), bilingual in a bilingual neighborhood, native son of its minority population and thus familiar with both cultures—he nevertheless betrays his patients, coworkers, and profession, not to mention his own people and neighbors. It's hard (impossible?) to gauge the medical damage and suffering his ethical lapses are causing.

Lenny is soon relieved of his duties and barred from ever working for our health department. Mentally exhausted by this betrayal, I comfort myself by saying that this experience should help prevent a repeat in the future.

Regrettably, there will be several more Lennys during my nearly three decades as a venereal disease control officer, all detected by improved quality control measures.

Eternal vigilance is a virtue even in a virtue-based profession.

(NS)

Rebuffed on the Rez

He's named as a sexual partner to a case of syphilis and lives on an Indian reservation in the Southwest.

Such reservations are legally sovereign polities, which is why it's a good idea for a public health official like me to check in with the tribal government before conducting official business on their turf. Because health matters are orchestrated by the tribal health center, it's decided that the clinic outreach worker, rather than I, be the person responsible for bringing him into the clinic.

He tests positive for syphilis, and is treated and interviewed for sexual partner information by the clinic outreach worker. He names an anonymous woman met at a powwow in another part of the state. Likely story, which I've heard before. Clearly this man does not want to identify his partners—and probably not to me either.

An arrangement is made on my behalf to talk with him offsite, a rendezvous he fails to attend. Another appointment follows. And another. Same discouraging outcome. This time, the clinic outreach worker resolutely promises that the patient will show up for the interview at the tribal health care center instead. The appointed time comes and goes, yet the result is the same. A half-hour later, the clinic phone

PART III: IN THE FIELD

rings; it's him and he asks if "the white guy" (me) is still waiting. Yes.

Not more than a minute later, the patient speeds by on his motorcycle, braids flying, and quickly disappears in a cloud of dust. I never see him again.

Chalk this one up in the "lose" column.

(TRE)

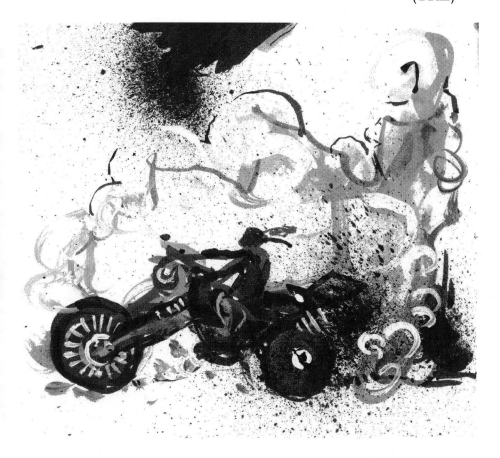

Do You Know Jack, Daniels?

When I receive a report of a positive syphilis test taken from a county jail inmate named Jack Daniels, I immediately suspect it's a phony name. Knowing from experience that people with something to hide often use aliases I jump to conclusions, not only inferring that he has a drinking problem, but that this problem may be fueled by an especial fondness for his favorite Kentucky bourbon, *Jack Daniels*.

Because neither his name nor birth date exists in our VD registry, I call the phone number he provides when booked in jail and, unsurprisingly, it's disconnected. All I have left is an address, which exists, but does not have a male resident, much less one named Jack. Having nothing to lose, I leave a note addressed to Jack Daniels in a sealed envelope and tell the resident to give it to him if he ever shows up. Two weeks later, I receive a phone call at my house late in the evening from a woman with a high-pitched voice resembling that of Miss Piggy's. She says her name is Marissa and that someone says I need to talk to her. I ask who that someone is, and Marissa gives me the address where I left the note. She explains that she used to be Jack but is now

Marissa. Eureka! (Now I also know why her voice sounds like Miss Piggy's!)

I explain that she has a positive test for syphilis and needs follow-up. Marissa then provides me with the (presumably real) name and birth date "she" uses at the time of his syphilis diagnosis a few years ago. The information matches. Case closed.

(NS)

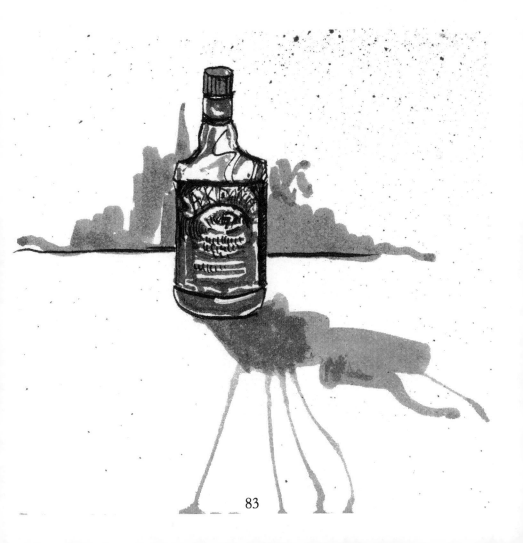

The Prisoner of Bel-Air

I enter the cavernous mansion occupied by one of television's well-known actors. People (and I am not one of them, for I seldom watch TV) familiar with his work praise his engaging on-screen personality.

I'm here because, earlier in the day, I call to tell him he's been exposed to syphilis. Distressed, he requests that I appear in person to confirm my identity as a health department official and provide further details about his putative exposure. It's not his engaging personality that greets me, but rather, a pro forma polite, understandably anxious one. While answering his questions, he nervously ambulates and I follow. I note the cold, impersonal feel of his sparsely-furnished interiors but am not very surprised, because I know he's single and living alone.

He asks for my age and tells me that I remind him of Ben Gazzara. He says he's interested in getting together. I tell him I'm married, flattered by his invitation, but personally and professionally not at liberty to accept.

It occurs to me that being well-known makes it difficult for him to find male partners while simultaneously protecting privacy and reputation—and that living alone in this huge, impersonal mansion, compounds what must be deep feelings of alienation.

If he indeed is engaging on screen, I think I understand why. He compensates.

(**JJP**)

The Geography of Risk

The risk of being exposed to VD is commonly thought to be random (at least for the non-monogamous). It takes only a few months of sexual partner tracing for VD sleuths like me to abandon this view as, surprisingly, many outings to locate exposed partners wind up in the same neighborhoods and, often, in the same buildings. VD transmissions tend to be clustered (cloistered?) events.

In my city there are two places where you're at high risk to get VD If you live at the pink house with a pinball machine on the front porch, your venereal disease risk is gonorrhea; if you live in the tall brick apartment building across the tracks a short distance away, it's syphilis.

In fact, given someone's name as a contact to syphilis whose domicile is unknown, my first move is to check the names listed on the apartment building's mailboxes, as this tactic often succeeds.

Clustering happens, because people often choose sexual partners from their own (sub)neighborhoods: the Temple of the Familiar. Cloistered indeed.[2]

(JJP, NS)

Apartment #505

Sexually transmitted diseases are not randomly or evenly distributed in society. Cases are often concentrated within specific age categories, in specific ethnic or racial groups, within specific sexual networks, and even in specific neighborhoods. It's not fair, but it's reality.

Syphilis is a case in point. In Denver during the mid-1980s, for example, most cases are being diagnosed

---

[2] Definition of "cloistered" used = separated from the world.

in gay or bisexual men. Darren is a thirty-year-old single man just diagnosed by his private doctor as having first-stage syphilis (a sore on his penis). The case is assigned to me for counseling and for the sexual partner interview.

Darren claims to be exclusively heterosexual and names, as the sole sexual partner during the period he acquires the infection, a woman he meets in a local bar. He doesn't remember Connie's last name, can't find her phone number, and doesn't know what she does or where she works. Likely story. He mentions that she lives in apartment #505 in a large apartment complex and provides a physical description. I remain skeptical and inclined to suspect that his sexual partner(s) are men. None of the standard interview motivations I use to get him to change his story and admit to having male partners yields any different result. He sticks by his story.

I visit the apartment complex, notice her name (which now includes a last name) on the mailbox, and knock on the door. No reply. The knock sounds hollow, as if the apartment is empty. The manager confirms that Connie has just moved. Encouraged that Darren is telling me the truth, I obtain a forwarding address from the post office and send the report to my public health colleagues in Washington State. She's located, examined, and treated for second-stage syphilis (a generalized rash).

This case reminds me that all bets are off when predicting individual behavior using population-level information.

(SKR)

I Know How to Make It Hard[3]

We're in a trailer park near a military base, where life is hard and children grow up quickly, especially in the absence of soldier fathers. "We" are a team of VD sleuths and child protection services workers.

A 4-year-old boy has gonorrhea, diagnosed at the military hospital after he tells his mother that his penis is burning and dripping. Although he denies sex play, his mother reveals that, a few days before his symptoms, she saw him hastily putting his pants

---

[3] Potterat JJ, Markewich GS, King RD, et al. Child-to-child transmission of gonorrhea: report of asymptomatic infection in a boy. *Pediatrics* 1986; 78: 711–712.

back on, in the company of a similarly occupied 5-year-old neighbor girl, in the trailer park's laundry room. On examination, this young girl has vaginal discharge (yes, positive for gonorrhea) and a recent history of burning on urination. Initially denying sex play, she eventually admits to having sex with the 4-year-old and with a 7-year-old neighbor boy. In turn, this boy is examined and, although symptomless, the gonorrhea culture is positive. After persistent prodding by the nurse, he tells her that "a long time ago" he was approached by the 5-year-old girl who, pointing to his groin, said that she knew "how to make it hard and what to do with it." He says sex took place in the crawl space underneath a neighbor's trailer several months ago.

Her mother's boyfriend, a 20-year-old soldier who shows no symptoms, denies contact with the child but tests positive for gonorrhea (as does the mother). At long last, the child finally admits that the soldier had sex with her and had "hurt me and will hurt me worse if she ever told anyone."

(HPZ, JJP)

All in the Family

Travis is 8 years old. His father brings him to the family physician, saying that Travis has pus coming out of his urethra and that it hurts when he pees. Travis says his symptoms appear after bumping against the school's playground equipment.

The urethral culture shows that Travis has gonorrhea. The physician calls me—the sole infectious disease investigator in this rural community—to request my presence during Travis's follow-up visit. I'm given use of a private room for as long as I need it. Travis insists he hurt himself on the playground but I, with some difficulty, convince him that gonorrhea infection occurs on another kind of playground. He finally admits to sex with someone but is bound by a promise not to tell. After half an hour of sitting quietly, and my assurance that he will not be hurt by telling me who that person is, he tells of sex with his older sister, a late teen who is later shown to be infected with gonorrhea, as is her boyfriend. Because of what the physician knows about the family (confidential and not revealed to me), he decides that the entire family be treated for gonorrhea. Unfortunately, no culture specimens are collected.

Although adults with sexually transmitted disease are shielded by confidentiality provisions from having their identity revealed to sexual partners, this legal protection does not apply to children. In this case, Child Protective Services intervenes and places Travis in foster care.

(TRE)

"I Didn't Know You Was Gay!"

A high-ranking Army sergeant, recently retired, is referred to me, the post dermatologist, because of a rash all over his body. Although I immediately spot it as secondary syphilis, it doesn't cross my mind that he got it homosexually, the way most syphilis cases in men are presently (the 1970s) acquired. Not only is he married, but everybody knows there are no homosexuals in this man's Army!

I also moonlight in the local health department's VD clinic and, as part of my epidemiological training, am invited to visit local prostitute hangouts ("the stroll") and gay bars, because they host high-risk populations.

Tonight, after clinic, my health department host and I are sitting in the town's largest gay bar, nursing a beer and learning to read this (for me) new environment. As we speak comes this self-same retired sergeant, who slaps me on the back and gleefully says: "I didn't know you was gay!"

It turns out that he's well known in the local gay community, because his wife and he take in stray gay men, usually servicemen, who need a safe and relaxing place to spend weekends, away from the military.

(GSM)

Queen Guinevere or Lancelot?

It's just before ten on Saturday night. At the invitation of the owners, I'm in the most popular gay bar in town—not as venereal disease control officer, but as curious guest. It's packed with patrons, and I can feel the excitement of the coming attraction, a campy and daring (I'm told) show by gay-circuit drag queens.

PART III: IN THE FIELD

It's my first drag queen show, and I mingle with them backstage, making small talk and probably asking stupid questions about costumes and role-playing, which they indulgently tolerate.

I'm particularly intrigued by the effeminate young man with florid manners and a lisp bordering on parody who calls himself Lancelot. I ask, within earshot of the other queens, why he chooses Lancelot when, given his craft and gender impersonations, he perhaps should more appropriately use Queen Guinevere.

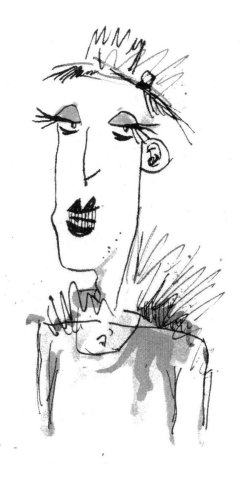

"Because of my love life; you see, I get lanced a lot!"

Mirth all around.

(JJP)

No, He Didn't Do It!

This incident features three different people: he's Hispanic, she's black, and I'm white. Each of us is in our twenties. He's been exposed to HIV, she's his fiancée, and I'm the visibly pregnant health department VD contact tracer.

It's a hot summer's day and I climb three flights of stairs to reach the apartment door. Now beet-red from the climb in this stifling apartment building, I knock on the door. She presently opens it, sees my red face, maternity clothes, and big belly and evidently reaches the wrong conclusion. She appears ready to pounce. I immediately blurt out: "No, he didn't do it!" This breaks the ice and we both start laughing. She invites me in.

As I privately inform him of his exposure to HIV he blanches, realizing that if and when he has to tell his fiancée (depending on the test result), she'll probably pounce. And certainly not laugh.

(HLR)

Gunorrhea Scare

I'm a contact tracer in VD clinic. My job is to confidentially find the sexual partners of people with venereal disease and refer them to medical care. I'm presently concentrating my efforts on snuffing out a raging gonorrhea outbreak in five local crack cocaine gangs.

I'm white, thirty, and long-haired, while most gang members (and wannabes) are black, about a decade younger than I, and clean-cut. My game plan is to convince both gangsters and hangers-on, which include very young and ethnically diverse women, that I'm not a cop, but an employee of the health department who can be trusted not to snitch. I routinely show up at places where gangsters and their friends congregate, such as hamburger joints, movie theaters, malls, clubs, and bars. "See and Be Seen" is my approach. Occasionally, gang members tail my car to determine my destination: friendly or hostile? And once, a gang leader invites me into an apartment stacked with illegal property—a mountain of cocaine and an arsenal of weapons and explosives—presumably to test my avowed neutrality.

I'm now trusted and rarely feel uncomfortable or threatened in gang social spaces. Yet there comes the day when the unexpected blindsides me. A mistrusting 14-year-old wannabe pulls a gun on me. With no time to think, I luckily defuse the situation by admiring the gun and asking for permission to hold it. Permission granted.

Now back to taming the gonorrhea outbreak, which is accomplished within a year. And both gonorrhea and gunorrhea scares become a footnote in Colorado Springs public health history.

(**SQM, Anonymous**)

Bad Blood

I'm a student in nursing school presently doing a rotation in the local health department. The program is intended to provide some experience with community medicine and field outreach. I'm supposed to be teamed with a trained public health nurse, but this time I'm doing a visit to a family with a premature infant all by myself.

I knock on the door. When it opens, a tall black man is angrily pointing a gun at me. Startled, if not terrified, I quickly explain the reason for my visit: to assess the baby's health and developmental milestones, as well as to see how the mother is doing. He lowers the gun and tells me not to mention "Bad Blood" under any circumstances.

It's mid-20th century in the Rocky Mountain region, and I've not yet heard of "Bad Blood". I learn later that it's a commonly-used term for syphilis in black communities, especially in the South where the family is from. From a medical point of view, the visit is successful, as both mother and baby are doing well.

Back at the health department where I summarize today's visit, I'm told that the nuclear family consists of the man, who is a pimp, the mother, who is a street prostitute, and the newborn, and that both adults are being treated for syphilis. The baby is, fortunately, not infected.

None of this information is provided prior to my visit, and this baptism under fire teaches me a crucial lesson: to collect as much social information on any patient I'm due to visit. I'm willing to bet that such a precaution will help prevent unwelcome surprises in the field, not to mention bad blood in the nursing department.

(HPZ)

Mankind, Meankind

Kind. Mean. Opposites. The world has its share of both kinds of people. And we public health workers, who reach out in various neighborhoods to locate the partners of people diagnosed with venereal disease, are not immune from being exposed to behavioral opposites.

I'm presently looking for a young woman whose lover, recently diagnosed with gonorrhea in our VD clinic, tells me she's likely to be home at this time of day. A young woman myself, I'm conscious of the potential danger in this poverty-stricken neighborhood. I park my car a few houses from my destination. No sooner done than a voice coming from a group of young people sitting on a porch tells me that I can't park in front of this house. I reply that the sign on the curb clearly allows free parking for up to two hours today and immediately proceed to the young woman's house. I return a few minutes later and notice that

PART III: IN THE FIELD

the curbside rear tire on my car is flat. Not a good sign.

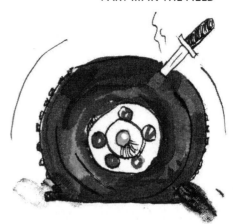

Because the youths on the porch are laughing at, and heckling, me as I inspect the tire, I decide not to encourage further mean spiritedness by changing the tire here. To minimize damage to the rim, I drive gingerly to a safer place about a block away, grateful that it was only one tire that was deflated. A wizened old man notices my distress and volunteers to help. He telephones the Automobile Association and keeps me company until the tire is fixed. The job done, I thank him for his kindness, telling him how it instantly changed my mood from dark to light.

As I drive away, I reflect on how easily acts of kindness can restore my (occasionally undermined) faith in mankind.

Mankind yes, Meankind no. What a difference one little letter makes!

(NS)

Hell Street Blues

Dontae, an adolescent, lives at home with his mother. His health is of concern, because he's named as the only sexual partner of a teenager with a raging pelvic infection caused by gonorrhea. Donna and I, in our twenties and white, are STD contact tracers with the health department. We're walking up the front steps of his home and knock on the door. A middle-aged black woman opens the door. I greet her and ask to speak to Dontae. The woman informs us that she's his mother, breathlessly demanding to know why we need to see him. I explain that this is a health matter, that he certainly is not in trouble, and that I plan to encourage him to discuss it with her, whereupon she screams: "You're on my property and I have a right to ask you motherfuckers these questions". (Colorado Statutes protect the confidentiality of sexual medical information of pre-adults.) Assuming that Dontae is not at home, I provide her with a sealed envelope containing my business card, asking her to please make sure he gets it.

That's when all hell breaks loose. The instant I proffer the envelope, she shoves me backwards from the door. Thinking that she's acting impulsively and probably regretting her aggressive behavior, I thank her and start to walk down the front steps. At that very moment, she sics her two teen daughters on us, all the while screaming multiple "motherfuckers!" at us. Donna is punched in the head by one girl, while the other jumps on my back, giving me a similar beating. I think about how long a head-beating might take before you get a concussion, all the while resolving to race for the safety of my car. Donna, a tall and solidly-built former college varsity athlete, pulls the girl away from me and I make it to the car. Meanwhile, the two girls are using a garden hose and a steel pipe to continue beating Donna. From the car, I scream her name, begging her to get in, which she presently does.

With torn clothes and emerging bruises, we drive to the nearest police station and file assault charges against the mother and her daughters. The police take photographs of us with our shredded blouses and scrapes. We go to the nearest emergency room to rule out serious injuries, while our supervisor notifies the Colorado Attorney General. The criminal justice system lets mother (two-year deferred judgment and sentencing for third degree assault, while under probation) off easy and daughters (no action taken) unscathed.

Fortunately, Donna and I escape serious injury. Police Sergeant Phil Esterhaus's concluding words at morning roll call in the television series *Hill Street Blues*—"Let's be careful out there"—now resonate and become our professional motto as well.

(**NS**)

What's the Way Out of Here?

Graham has syphilis and I, a public health worker, need to interview him for sexual partner information. Relaxed and friendly on the phone, he suggests meeting in person at his apartment, which I know to be in a decent neighborhood.

As I walk up to the door and knock, neither my built-in female caution nor gut feeling portends danger. A man opens the door and I ask to speak to Graham. "He'll be right out", says he. Graham invites me in. The house is very dark, spooky even. Because there are others in the house, he suggests talking in his bedroom, which features only a mattress on the floor and a chair, on which sits a (crack?) pipe. And yes, the room is thick with smoke. He asks me to sit on the chair, himself choosing to lay on the mattress.

I don't frighten easily, but this is different. In what way, I don't really know. Of all the "shady" places I've visited during my 27 years as a VD contact tracer never have I been as frightened by my patients' surroundings as at Graham's, and I've been to many dubious places. And never in my career of doing VD interviews have I done one as quickly; this despite the fact that Graham is chatty and I constantly struggle to keep him on task.

The way out of here is concentration and, above all, speed.

(TRM)

Hurricane Mama

Locating the right apartment in this dilapidated neighborhood is challenging, but I finally succeed. I'm looking for Tamika, 13 years old, whose gonorrhea and chlamydia tests are positive in VD clinic, where I work as a contact tracer. My conversation with Tamika, woman to woman (as it were), is uneventful, and I leave with her promise to be in clinic tomorrow afternoon.

Tamika's mother (I later learn), who is not at the door at the time of our conversation, sees me leave and, all of a sudden and apparently out of nowhere, bulldozes down the sidewalk, hot breath and screams literally an inch from my face. Lots of cuss words. Threats of physical harm. Yet I manage to put on my best deer-in-the-headlights expression and somehow succeed well enough that Hurricane Mama backs down. Because I'm petite? Who knows?

It's also the last time I do a field visit to a teenager's home address. There's more than one way to avoid shrewish mothers.

(PM)

Exit Strategy

A bar is a good place to meet sexual partners. Hence, hardly a week goes by that I'm not visiting some bar looking for someone named as a contact to VD who's said to hang out there.

My fellow health department contact tracers and I also frequently go to bars or restaurants, to socialize after work and cement workplace camaraderie. Our job may be exotic, but it's also difficult, and often frustrating. Sharing success, as well as disappointing, stories is therapeutic, for it helps recharge our batteries. Our peculiar behavior emerges when we jockey for position at table. This behavior is based on professional habit. It resembles a game of musical chairs, as we circle the table several times for the best seat in the house; it's the one facing the door, because one needs a clear view of the exit in case one needs to leave quickly to avoid trouble.

Contact tracers in Detroit are taught to knock on the door and then quickly step aside, to avoid facing the muzzle of a gun between one's eyes. In Denver, we're taught to keep an eye on the door, not only to see comings and goings, but as an escape route in potentially charged situations.

Even today, a decade after my retirement from contact tracer duties, I continue to look for a seat at table with the clearest view of the front door.

Old habits, like exit strategies, die hard.

(NS)

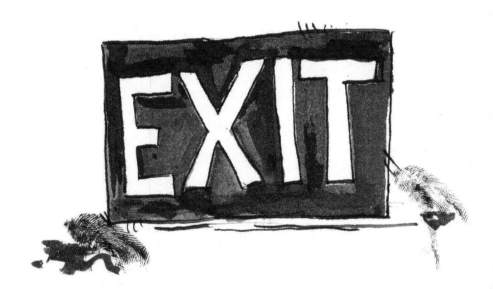

PART III: IN THE FIELD

Part IV: HIV/AIDS

This new and (initially) invariably fatal infection took America by surprise in the early 1980s, leaving an indelible footprint in the universe of sexually transmissible diseases.

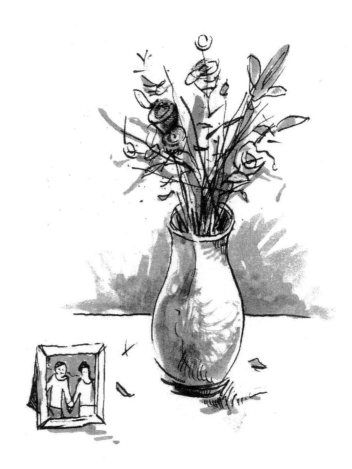

HIV Testing and Murphy('s Law)

It's 1986, five years since the AIDS epidemic is identified. Local pastors, much like the Reagan Administration, are mostly silent about this new plague. A newly-ordained Catholic priest, whose core commitment is to pastoral care for pariahs and those on the margins of society ("True Catholic values", he tells me) contacts us at the health department. He wants to know how he can help relieve some of the anxiety and suffering of those at high risk for HIV.

First things first. He volunteers to experience the required counseling and testing procedure, so that he can confidently recommend this anxiety-laden visit to his constituents. We are pleased, because our test site has operated successfully for a year and has an unblemished record of treating patients with compassion and dignity. Moreover, our logistics are perfect; for example, we've never lost a test specimen.

There is a first time for everything. Whose blood test specimen is lost in transit to the laboratory? You guessed it. And (before this fact is known) who's put through the (repeat) anxiety of learning that the test result is not back within a week as promised ("What's wrong with my blood"?), or within 10 days, or even 14?

It's a true measure of his compassionate character that he forgives us our trespasses and becomes a founding member of the local AIDS prevention and care organization.

A Franciscan pastor, this Father Murphy.

(RR)

Intimate Diseases

I'm driving to keep an appointment with Freddie at his apartment. I'm working in the sexually transmitted diseases program of our health department and, because his internist tells me he's a newly diagnosed case of HIV, I'm on my way to interview him for sexual partner information. The doctor tells me he's a 22-year-old gay man.

He answers the door wearing a T-shirt and shorts. As soon as I see him, I notice a rash on both legs and ask him how long it's been there. He answers: "A short while" and tells me he's being treated for eczema. I've been a nurse for more than three decades and immediately know it's secondary (the rash stage) syphilis. After the interview, I recommend that he be blood tested to confirm my rash (pun intended) judgment, which he does and which comes back positive for syphilis.

From the earliest days (early 16th century) syphilis rashes are known to resemble other conditions, which is why physicians call it "The Great Imitator". And so what is it that makes me virtually certain that Freddie's rash is syphilis and not some other disease? Recent information from the medical literature indicates that a large proportion of men with HIV also have concurrent syphilis infection, and vice-versa. This is what gives me confidence bordering on cockiness.

Two dreaded sexually transmitted diseases are now known to be intimately connected.

When I think about it: how unsurprising!

(HPZ)

Cruising the Sexual Superhighway

Stan is a personable and outgoing man in his early 40s being tested for HIV in our health department clinic. He volunteers to participate in a study about how people remember their sexual partners. The ultimate goal is to develop effective interviewing techniques to obtain more complete recall. (See "Magnetic" on page 34 as an example.)

I've interviewed hundreds of STD patients who reveal unusual and even exotic details about their sex lives, yet Stan amazes me with the scope of his sexual adventurism and uncanny memory. In just 20 minutes, he happily rattles off the names of the 112 male partners he's had sex with during the last dozen months—sampling these men in 19 different cities sprinkled across 7 American states and 3 Canadian provinces. Some of these men hailed from yet other states and countries.

Stan seemingly has radar for fun partners. For example, one of his partners he meets using his CB radio, while another is an anonymous motorist with whom he "plays" following a spontaneous game of tag on the freeway. From a public health perspective,

Stan's vivid accounts highlight the global sexual network that facilitates rapid STD transmission among gay men.

Yet I can't help thinking that many straight men would kill to live the heterosexual equivalent of Stan's sex life.

(DDB)

Too Good-Looking to be Real

This young man is exceptionally good-looking, and the nurses, including me, in our sexually transmitted diseases clinic, notice his beauty right away. He's here to find out the result of the HIV test he took a week ago.

The test is positive, and he absorbs the shock of this disturbing news (seemingly too) well. After explaining its significance and counseling him about safer behaviors and the importance of conscientious medical follow-up, I ask him about his sexual partners during the preceding year. Without hesitation he names twelve different women for that period. (Sort of a "Woman of The Month Casanova", I secretly think.)

The twelve "different" women are not at all different: one after the other is now being described as a tall, gorgeous, blonde-haired (down to her waist, of course), blue-eyed stunner. He recalls the first name of only half of these out-of-this-world beauties and knows none of their last. It takes little time for me to realize that this is a fabrication; these girls are just too good looking to be real. Moreover, because he has HIV, he's likelier to be gay than straight. My next question is: "OK. Now that we've talked about the girls, let's talk about the men you're having sex with". "What makes you think that?" he asks.

"What makes me think that" turns out to be common knowledge: if a man is too good-looking to be real, he's likelier to be gay than straight. At least that's our nurses' experience, after decades of carefully observing patients in our STD clinic. As some wise doctor once said: "The keen clinical eye misses nothing".

And so begins his listing of a dozen sexual partners, all (different) men.

(HPZ)

PART IV: HIV / AIDS

It's Condom Sense

He's a newly-ordained priest and his focus is on the disenfranchised and demonized.

It's also early in the AIDS epidemic, and many young people, especially those on the margins of society, are dying of sex. He wants to help prevent this deadly syndrome among his parishioners but, for various reasons, the Church opposes use of condoms. Although violating official doctrine is anathema, he resolves that saving lives is paramount. The stubborn fact is that this disease kills, and kills quickly. There is, therefore, no time to lose or to argue the fine print of theology.

He appears on local radio programs advocating a menu of sexual self-defense strategies—from abstinence, to monogamy, to safer practices, to use of barrier protections such as condoms. A priestly profile in courage.

When I ask him to explain himself, he answers that it's simply common sense, something that is bound to result in less suffering than (often intractable) ideology.

It makes condom sense to me as well.

(RR)

Analomy?

She tests positive for HIV on a U.S. Army pre-induction physical. A Spanish speaker whose command of English is modest, she brings her aunt to the interview to help translate. She names three sexual partners, including her heroin-injecting husband who, though found to be HIV-positive in another state, does not inform her. What puzzles her is how she could have gotten infected, for not only does she deny ever injecting drugs, but confesses to seldom having vaginal sex. A potential anomaly indeed.

Trying to understand her sexuality, I ask why. She hesitatingly starts to relate her inability to achieve orgasm from "straight up" intercourse but, suddenly animated, she heads to the bedroom to fetch her sex toys; she then excitedly (via her aunt's translation, of course) reveals that anal insertion is what she needs to achieve orgasm, all the while exhibiting her extensive collection of dildos, butt plugs, and anal beads.

PART IV: HIV / AIDS

So much for our failure as public health messengers to clearly and persistently emphasize the dangers of unprotected anal sex in heterosexual populations, for it now seems readily apparent how she acquired HIV. A real analomy indeed.

(SQM, Anonymous)

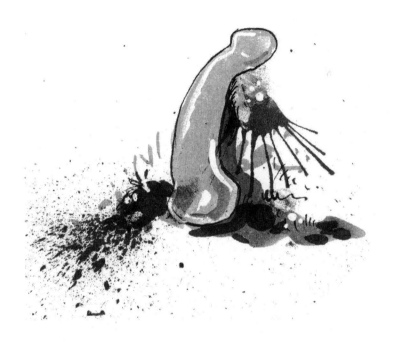

Get Rid of Smut

1986. Early autumn. The crescendo of concern surrounding the recent prediction by various (usually self-appointed) pundits that AIDS is about to cross over into the heterosexual population ("The Second Wave of the Epidemic") is why we're empanelled in a local television studio. "We" are a motley group of stakeholders, ranging from representatives of district schools, Christian churches, the health department (me) and, predictably for Colorado Springs, one ideologically motivated funny-mentalist with an Anti-Smut Agenda (anti-homosexual, anti-nonmatrimonial sex, anti-adult bookstore, anti-prostitution, anti-pornography, anti-...). Excepting the Catholic priest who non-judgmentally offers pastoral care to homosexuals (read: pariahs), there is no spokesperson from our gay communities.

Comes the time, midway through the televised discussion, when the anti-smut purveyor graphically describes his visit to a local adult bookstore, where "filthy" private booths host furtive sex between presumably heterosexual married men and bisexual/gay men. In his word: cesspools. He criticizes the health department for failing to shut down such an establishment, complaining that unprotected exposure to the various sex-derived body fluids contaminating the floors could infect someone.

Thus spake the health department representative: "Surely you don't go in there barefooted, do you?"

(JJP)

High School Confidential

I dislike bullies, and have as far back as kindergarten. Maybe it's my female protective instincts. It's the mid-1970s as I enter high school and the bullying seems to escalate every new school year. Even though I'm diminutive, I find myself forcefully defending a half-dozen timid male classmates who are targets of bullying. I've known them since elementary school and yes, a few are neighbors.

Fast forward ten years. I'm now a contact tracer for the health department's HIV control program. Presently I'm looking for Martin, who's being named as a sexual partner to an AIDS case. (He's a boy who really liked me in high school, but we never dated.) I arrive at his apartment. No one answers the bell. I leave a note asking him to call me as soon as he can about a personal matter, signing my full name, including a smiley face.

Martin calls a few hours later, sounding excited at what he (mis)construes as a prospective date. It pains me to inform him of his exposure to AIDS and pains me even more to inform him, ten days later, that he's HIV-positive. On interview he names sexual partners of both sexes and it suddenly dawns on me that the bullying may be due to perceived homosexuality.

End of story?

Regrettably no. During the next four years, five other victims of bullying in my high school class are diagnosed with HIV infection. All are gay men. Which also, to me, unfortunately explains the bullying.

(HLR)

If Asked, Don't Tell

It's early in the epidemic, and doctors at Walter Reed Army Hospital are reporting that AIDS-virus positive soldiers are acquiring the infection heterosexually, unlike their civilian counterparts who acquire it homosexually. They blame prostitutes for infecting the soldiers, an assertion unencumbered by evidence other than hearsay.

Because our sexually transmitted diseases control program works closely with our local military installations, we ask permission to interview their

AIDS patients to see if soldiers report different risk factors to civilian than to military interviewers. Our experience tells us that people rarely reveal pejorative personal information to employers and that soldiers are also unlikely to do so with their employer.

It takes fewer than two dozen interviews to show that risk factors revealed to civilian and military interviewers differ radically. Risks for soldiers mirror those in civilian communities: about 70% of cases occur in men who have sex with men, and 15% in street-drug injectors (the rest have undetermined factors). This reminds us that soldiers are civilians wearing uniforms and that if asked by military authorities, they probably won't tell[4].

(JJP, LP)

19,000 to 1 Odds

Clarence is a middle-aged, never married, highly placed public servant recently diagnosed with AIDS by his private doctor. It's early in the epidemic, and Clarence fits the current picture of the stereotypic

---

[4] Potterat JJ, Phillips L, Muth JB. Lying to military physicians about risk factors for HIV infections. *Journal of the American Medical Association* 1987; 257: 1727.

AIDS patient in North America: white, middle class, educated, and homosexual.

Because I'm well-known locally as a sexually transmitted diseases investigator, he insists on discussing AIDS exposure information in a discreet location. There, he tells me that he often travels to the Caribbean—specifically Haiti—to relax, and that he likely picked up this virus from a Haitian prostitute. My reaction: convenient, cop-out explanation. Not only do I know that older North American gay men frequently travel to the Caribbean to pick up young locals at bargain prices, but that his explanation is unlikely to account for other positive blood tests done by his doctor: hepatitis-B (HBV) and cytomegalovirus (CMV). At least he's providing some truthful information: where he likely picks up infection and by what means; it's just that I think he's reporting the wrong sex for his sexual partner(s). Yet no amount of motivational coaxing or ironclad guarantees of confidentiality (even vis-à-vis his doctor) applied during nearly two hours of discussion makes him recant.

What does finally make him change his story is the last card I play. I scribble, on the back of a paper napkin, the mathematical probability of a heterosexual person having all 3 blood markers (AIDS, HBV, CMV) combined: 0.000008 (8 out of 1,000,000), whereas in a homosexual man, the combined proportion is 0.15 (15 out of 100), for a difference in odds of triple infection of nearly 19,000 to 1.[5]

Patients may lie, but blood doesn't.

(JJP)

Hoping Against Hope

Keith is in his early 40s and has just tested for HIV in our public health clinic. It's a good thing he does, because he's recently been exposed to HIV. After hearing about our study on how people recall their sex partners, he volunteers to participate.

Although affable, he's clearly distressed when talking about his sexual partners. He confides that most

---

[5] This mathematical argument is considered worthy of dissemination and appears in Potterat JJ, Muth JB, Markewich GS. Serological markers of sexual orientation in AIDS-virus infected men. *Journal of the American Medical Association* 1986; 256: 712.

take advantage of him. His trusting nature repeatedly puts him in danger, as he's a prostitute, servicing both men and women.

Some of his male clients are HIV-positive but nevertheless engage him in very high-risk sex, such as unprotected anal intercourse. One recently tricked him, claiming to have used a condom when, in fact, he didn't. His other male clients are mentally ill, alcoholic, drug-addicted, and/or physically abusive.

Keith tells me he's even suffered multiple attempted or completed rapes by clients and other men. One client rapes him at gunpoint. Another time, he goes to a restroom to relieve himself and is sodomized by a stranger in a surprise attack.

Keith often does things professionally that make him uncomfortable, particularly when he tries to accommodate client fantasies. For example, he endures bondage, receives oral sex from a demanding woman in an outdoor parking lot, has vaginal sex with a woman half his age who wants his baby (he withdraws before ejaculation), and has sex with disgusting clients, such as an aggressive woman who reeks of unbearable body odor.

Being optimistic, Keith vows that from now on he'll accept only safe, sane and sober clients who share his values (family values in particular, ironically enough). To my ears, it sounds like he's hoping against hope.

(DDB)

Not Investigated Rigorously (N.I.R.)

The national Centers for Disease Control classifies AIDS cases by major risk factor, such as male homosexuality, injecting drug use, or blood transfusion, and also by risk marker, such as Haitian origin. When a newly-reported case reaches the local health department with none of the known risk categories checked it's categorized as N.I.R. (No Identified Risk). It's our job as infectious disease sleuths to contact the medical facility making the report to find out if the missing information is an oversight or if the risk category is truly unknown. That's the passive approach and the one most often used by health departments, especially when there are many N.I.R. cases. Since it's usually done by telephone in the comfort of your office, it can be viewed as the lazy AIDS epidemiologist's approach.

The active approach is to locate the AIDS patient and do a thorough, painstaking interview in person in a private place. This takes time, effort and, above all, skill and perseverance. It's what we choose to do and our experience shows that the vast majority of cases initially classified as N.I.R. can be reclassified, after conscientious follow-up, into one or more of the previously known risk categories. Such accuracy is critical for the proper allocation of our limited control and prevention energies.

And so, it's not that N.I.R. points to new, yet to be defined modes of transmission. Our experience indicates that N.I.R. really should stand for "Not Investigated Rigorously".

(JJP)

Down-Low

Being African-American, I know about homophobia in black communities, and I also know how hard it is to be black, straight or gay. There, being gay and living the gay life is viewed as a white, effeminate phenomenon. In a culture where masculinity is highly-prized, open homosexuality is to be avoided, and hence, the wise strategy for black men practicing homosexual acts is to remain closeted. Not to do so is to risk social isolation, discrimination, and verbal or physical abuse. Black men who have sex with men keep the appearance of heterosexuality, even having sex with, or being married to, women. To avoid using labels from the white world, they refer to this deception as living on the "Down-low".

Today, two African-American men come to our clinic requesting to be tested for sexually transmitted diseases and HIV. They tell me that they've recently moved to Colorado Springs aiming for a fresh start away from the East Coast. Their relationship has been rocky ever since another man in New York City entered the picture, and they want to be sure everything is OK before resuming monogamous sexual relations.

To prepare them for the worst I tell them that, being from the Down-low in New York City, the probability of being HIV-positive is high. A week later, the tests confirm my fears: both men have HIV infection.

When I inform them, the news hits them hard. They ask me, a heterosexual married black man, if I have any idea "how hard it is to be black *and* homosexual *and* hiding the Down-low secret from our families for many years". I answer that I can only try to imagine what it feels like: "Down low".

(**DLG**)

Sexual Boundaries, Anyone?

He's a 28-year-old man, and I'm a woman about his age. He's a patient in the local VD clinic and has just tested positive for HIV. It's my job to notify him and to find out from whom he acquired infection and to whom he may have transmitted it. He lives in his grandparents' basement apartment, where we meet for our private consultation.

His test result neither shocks nor panics him. To get a sense for how long he's been infected, I start with the usual questions about symptoms: weight loss, night sweats, diarrhea, swollen glands, cough, fatigue, and skin eruptions. He tells me he has the "opposite of diarrhea". Puzzled, I ask for clarification, at which point he reaches into his nightstand drawer, withdraws a large dildo, and explains that "I'm so plugged up, I can't get this up my ass". As for skin eruptions he, wearing only sweatpants, suddenly whips them down and shows me what looks like a paper cut on his penis.

I know now that this is not going to be a normal interview. Indeed, he's not done with his penis. He begins to masturbate, intently watching my reaction—as I'm sitting on his bed. Shocked, yet struggling to remain nonjudgmental (as we are trained to be), I immediately stand up, letting him know that there's a time and place for everything, but that this was hardly either. I tell him that I will return with a colleague to complete these procedures. I ask him how likely he's to be here next week and he tells me "unlikely".

Refusing to admit on initial interview that, among sexual partners other than his girlfriend, are men, he readily discusses his homosexual contacts with my (male) colleague two weeks later, apologizing to me for initially withholding this information. Among his sexual partners he lists his older (by ten years) brother, now dead of AIDS. Among other questions, he's asked about the age of the youngest person he's had sex with, to which he replies: "my cousin; he was 13". Nothing about his demeanor or facial expressions betrays any sense that what he's done is in any way wrong.

Upon subsequent medical examination he, his male partner, and girlfriend are all diagnosed with early syphilis. Of named sexual partners, only his brother is known to have had, like him, HIV infection.

(**Anonymous**)

Nasty, Brutish, and Short

On the same day that I visit the HIV-positive man featured in the previous vignette, I prepare to visit an HIV-positive woman in mid-pregnancy. As I approach her apartment building, I'm stunned by the sight of children with a shopping cart, two of whom are in it sitting on a case of beer, being pushed by an 8- to 10-year-old drinking a beer. The children in the cart are 3–5 years old and one of them is also drinking a beer. What to do, this being another "normal" day on the streets.

I keep walking, find the apartment, knock on the door. I'm greeted by a very (crack-cocaine induced?) thin woman with a softball-sized baby bump, holding an 8-month-old baby boy, with a two-and-a-half-year-old boy wrapped around her legs. She thinks I'm there to talk her into having an abortion, as the hospital staff has reportedly recommended. I reassure her that I'm here to help with her needs, as well as those of her exposed partners and children, all of whom should be tested for HIV.

She is very ill and tired. The baby has recurring diarrhea and there are no fresh diapers in the apartment. She uses the kitchen sink to rinse out the used disposable diaper, intending to replace this wet (and still dirty) diaper on the baby, using masking tape to secure it. While at the sink, she leaves the naked baby boy on his back on the floor, right in front of me, as the two-and-a-half-year-old boy plays with the baby's penis. Disturbed by this sight, I silently wag my finger at the child, shake my head emphatically, mouthing the word "No". (I don't want his mother to hear me reprimand her child, nor do I want to explain what I'm witnessing.) The little brat smiles at me and proceeds to redouble his efforts with his brother's penis. I wave my hand in front of his face to shoo him away from the baby. He leers at me, laughs, and resumes yanking, this time with greater vigor. As his mother returns from the kitchen, he stops yanking.

Where did the child learn this? I need to leave, especially as I'm having difficulty breathing. I get up and smooth the back of my jeans. I presently realize that my hand is soaking wet. Gross! Who knows what I sat on.

This is the day that I (almost) quit my job.

PS. Her pregnancy produces a daughter who dies at three weeks of age, and she herself dies 4 months later. Her two children test HIV-negative. Her HIV-positive husband remains alive twenty years later (at last check).

(Anonymous)

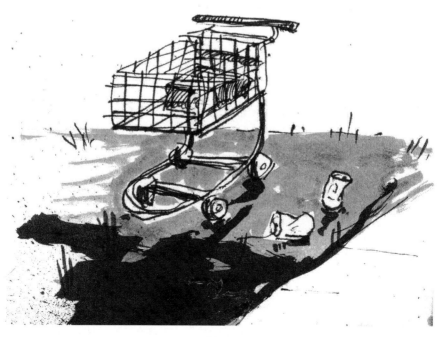

PART IV: HIV / AIDS

Of Mothers, Babies, HIV, and the Future

Even to this day, nearly thirty years later, I see her anxious eyes as she searches my face for answers. Tabitha is a young, HIV-positive mother with a newborn baby. Because HIV science is young, answers about HIV transmission risks and life expectancy are still foggy.

A newly-minted HIV contact tracer for the health department (and mother of young children myself), I do my best to comfort and reassure her. We're sitting on her living room floor while I emphasize how quickly new discoveries, especially treatments, are being made. She's still very scared, not to mention puzzled by my explanations of incubation periods, immune system cells, and sexual transmission risks. The baby continues to squirm in her blankets.

Tabitha is the first HIV-positive mother I counsel and, because her baby is a "contact" (via passage through the birth canal), a blood test is indicated. But how does one get blood from a two-inch foot? My experience with drawing bloods from contacts in the field is confined to adults, hence I decide to bundle mother and baby and drive to Denver's Children's

Hospital where a kind, gentle nurse pricks the howling baby's heel, squeezing two tiny glass tubes of blood. Mission accomplished.

Now comes the agonizing part: waiting for results, which takes days. But the wait ends positively, for the baby is not HIV-infected.

There are not many days when I don't wonder if Tabitha lives to see her baby reach maturity.

(AH)

Double Whammy

A physician in rural Colorado calls me, a health department HIV contact tracer, to ask for my help in notifying a Spanish-speaking patient of her positive prenatal HIV test. Not only does he not have any experience counseling HIV patients, but his command of Spanish is elementary. And there's one more thing I need to know, and he tells me of her recent miscarriage.

Consuelo and I meet a few hours later at her physician's office where, after introducing me and reassuringly (patronizingly?) patting her on the head, he arranges for a private room. She looks at me with a blank expression, which I interpret as sorrow. Apprehensively, given her recent loss, I tell her of her positive HIV test. Her face drops, agony replacing the blank stare. She cries. And cries. I try to calm her. The crying continues. She's inconsolable.

A half-hour later, as she begins to collect herself, I explain HIV infection and, above all, about how manageable this disease is given modern medicine. When we discuss sexual partners, she explains that she's only been married a few months, and resumes crying. Concerned about her husband, she asks if her infection also means he has it. I tell her it's an unknown until he's tested. She then asks me to tell him, and I inform her that, although I can be with her when she tells him, it's her job to do so.

I call her husband at work, tell him that Consuelo has a medical problem he needs to know about, and that it would be best if he came home. And home is where we meet when he learns the bad news. Crying and choking on her words, Consuelo finds the courage to tell him. Initially upset, shock is followed by lots of tears. Now both of them are crying a river. After spending 3 hours with them, not leaving until I feel they can cope, I go home. I rarely bring the vicissitudes of my work home, but in this case I cry for a solid 2 hours.

Her husband's HIV test returns negative a week later, and both are subsequently lost to follow-up. I thus don't learn of the longer-term impact of this double whammy.

(TRM)

Off His Meds

When contacting people who are named as sexual or drug-injecting partners of AIDS patients, I sometimes meet one who's clearly mentally ill. Bart is one of them. And today, is he ever a mess.

I knock on the door, which he soon opens. I tell him that I'm a nurse from the health department and need to talk with him in private. He looks terrible, as does his apartment, which is in complete shambles: broken chairs everywhere, tables and mattresses overturned, ripped curtains and dirty laundry on the floor, scattered broken lamps and dishes. I quickly assess the damage as self-inflicted vandalism, the product of an acute psychotic crisis.

Calmly, I ask if we can sit on the sole intact piece of furniture, a small bed, and softly say: "Do you take medicine?" "Yes". "Please show it to me". Bart brings it and I ask him to take it now, which he does. He even brings a glass of water for me (it's a very hot day) from one of the few remaining unbroken glasses! I'm touched and realize we're connecting. He tells me that voices are talking to him but seem to be fading. I continue talking with him, calming him. There's no point in telling him now about his possible exposure to AIDS, and so I ask if I can come back soon. He says: "Sure, you're keeping the voices from me. Thank you".

Back at the office a male coworker, anxious about my safety, insists that he accompany me on any return trip. We visit Bart a week later and, because he's on his meds, he's functioning well. The apartment is no longer a mess, as his landlord has replaced the broken furniture, lamps, and ripped curtains.

Bart fortunately tests negative for HIV.

(**HPZ, DEW**)

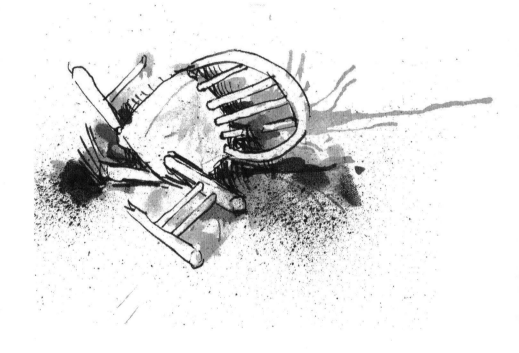

HIV Ending

When he arrives in clinic, my first impression is that he's an affable middle-aged man with boyish good looks and a ready smile. I'm intrigued, because he's so different from the kind of person usually seen in VD clinic. I also suspect his smile is forced. I'm thus especially curious about his reason for being here.

It takes no time for him to tell me that he wants to confirm he has AIDS. This is the no-nonsense, get-to-the-point statement I expect from an engineer, which he is. After finding out that he is living with his wife and teen-aged children, he reveals that she's having an affair with another man. I try to reassure him that being infected because of his wife's infidelity is extremely unlikely since HIV is very inefficiently transmitted during "normal" intercourse, especially vagina-to-penis. I tell him that even if his wife has HIV, his probability of acquiring it sexually would be in the range of about 1 chance in 3,000 per sex act, probably even much less (thinking that quantifying the risk would appeal to an engineer).

Ten days later, the test confirms his belief. Stunned by this improbable result, and accustomed to expecting white middle-aged men with HIV to have acquired it via sex with other men, I probe for such a history. He quickly stuns me again by saying that he deliberately sought infection as a means of ending life. Why HIV? Because, as a devout Catholic, he is not allowed to commit suicide. He then explains that his life has taken many turns for the worse in the last few years, from being terminated at his job, to losing his wife's affection, to being unable to secure new employment where his family wants to live, to raising problematic teenagers, and to suddenly and inexplicably feeling attracted to men. And this last reason is why he decides to visit gay bathhouses where, he learns from early newspaper accounts, HIV is rampant. After multiple episodes of unprotected receptive anal intercourse during a long holiday weekend, which occurs about six weeks ago, he comes to my clinic. Because these two visits occur at a time when AIDS is considered rapidly fatal, and certainly before any treatment is available to fight HIV, he no longer has any reason to attend. He disappears from our clinic roster and is lost to follow-up. It is thus the only HIV ending I can know.

(JJP)

Irresponsible Sex

When I think about their case, I visualize a spider trapping a fly. Shantae is the spider and Jose, the fly. They are 15-year-old lovers seeking HIV testing in VD clinic, where I work as a contact tracer. I tell them that they're at low risk for HIV unless they've engaged in unprotected receptive anal intercourse or are sharing HIV-contaminated equipment during injecting drug use, both of which activities they deny. Yet Shantae insists on their being tested. Her rapid screening test comes back positive within 20 minutes, as does Jose's. I'm stunned, given that neither 15-year-old admits to the high-risk behaviors usually associated with HIV infection in our county.

Upon confirmation of the rapid test's accuracy a week later, each is privately interviewed for additional risk information. Jose's story does not change. Shantae, on the other hand, reveals that both her parents are HIV-positive, and that she's been HIV-positive since birth without ever being sick. Shantae neither uses condoms during sex, nor informs Jose of her HIV status.

I'm livid: how could a girlfriend know she's HIV-positive and not inform her partner, so he can take defensive measures? How utterly irresponsible. (And she tells me that she wouldn't hurt a fly.)

Jose is confused, disoriented. I feel betrayed on his behalf. Above all, my heart goes out to him: so young to deal with such an undeserved burden.

The spider does hurt the fly. I'm left to wonder how many other men Shantae will irresponsibly expose during her sexually active years.

Moreover, I now realize that there are limits to my wanting to be non-judgmental.

(Anonymous)

No Identified Risk Interview

I'm in the home of a family whose son and daughter died of AIDS about a year ago. We're in a time when sibling HIV infections, and HIV infections and AIDS deaths in women are rare. Case overload prevents my health department from getting to all cases as rapidly as possible, but there's nevertheless continuing interest in identifying risk factors and, if possible, people exposed to the deceased. Unfortunately, neither item of public health interest is recorded in either their medical charts or in health department public health records.

During this "No Identified Risk" interview the parents reveal, among other leads, their daughter's fondness for a man named Mick who works at a liquor store in a principally African-American section of downtown Denver. When I reach it, it's not only closed but boarded up. Because I'm familiar with this area and my work occasionally takes me to a nearby local bar, I ask the bartender if he knows someone named Mick who works at a neighborhood liquor store. He doesn't. I ask his permission to leave a note in a sealed envelope in case he ever shows up or in case someone else knows him.

No sooner am I back in my office than the phone rings. It's Mick on the line! (Is Lady Luck on my side today or what?) I explain that he may, a long time ago, have been exposed to someone with AIDS and am interested in discussing his options. He agrees and I meet him in his neighborhood, counseling him and drawing his blood in my car.

Fortunately for him, his test comes back negative. Lady Luck was apparently on his side as well!

(SKR)

Interviewing the Dead

To identify risk factors and exposed partners of a person with AIDS I normally do the interview in person, in private. This is called a "contact interview"; its aim is to find out how and from whom the patient acquires infection (going upstream), and to whom it may be transmitted (downstream). Although straightforward in concept it's not easy to do, because a patient often presents obstacles and objections to this discovery process.

A contact interview may be difficult to do, but how does one interview a dead patient?

It's early in the AIDS epidemic, and we disease sleuths need to learn from every patient, even if dead by the time their case is reported to our health department. That's why the HIV post-mortem interview is invented. It consists of locating family and friends of the deceased to discreetly (respecting medical confidentiality as much as possible) identify likely risk factors and sexual partners.

This interviewing procedure is yet one more tool we can use to elucidate HIV transmission patterns and to warn people possibly exposed who could not ever be warned by their dead (ex-)partner.

Dead Souls (as Gogol knew) can make a difference.

(JJP, NS)

And Now, Kealani

It's late December, and I'm looking forward to the holiday party later this afternoon. But first I, a health department HIV contact tracer, need to review the hospital chart of a patient in his fifties whose HIV test is positive. At the time Kealani shows up at the emergency room, he has fever, diarrhea, and other flu-like symptoms. The medical advice is straightforward: go home, hydrate, and rest.

To inform him of his HIV test result and to interview him for the names of exposed sex or/and injecting-drug partners, I knock on the door of his apartment. Kealani opens it wearing only a hastily placed bath towel around his waist. He's disheveled, smells of feces, urine, and vomit. As he attempts to reach the sofa from whence he apparently rose, his frail, 90-pound body topples to the floor.

I help him up onto the sofa, now covered with soiled towels, where he's been nursing his illness. Shocking. Equally shocking are the thoughts that race through my mind. Is he going to die soon, right in front of me? Who do I call? And how am I ever going to interview Kealani for the necessary public health information?

I give him his test result and find out where his family is. I call for an ambulance, skip the holiday party, and visit him in his hospital room later that evening. He's unconscious, in multiple organ failure, and not expected to regain consciousness.

Family members arrive from out of state the next evening and, miraculously, Kealani is alert, eating, drinking, and even joking around. I'm even able to interview himfor risk factor and partner information, even as I struggle with the ethics of exercising my professional duties given his circumstances. Fortunately, he's very cooperative, which attenuates some of my guilty feelings.

On day 3, he dies. And now, Kealani ("Clear sky" in Hawaiian).

(PM)

PART IV: HIV / AIDS

The Birthday Card

Craig no longer has days, but only hours to live. His lover, Harold, musters the courage to call Craig's parents in a distant state, anxious about their relationship's defining characteristic: alienation. "Your son is dying of AIDS, and there's not much time if you want to see him before he dies." Over the telephone line, Harold can feel the tension, the anger even.

A few hours later, Craig's father calls and says that they are not coming. The family priest has assured them that because Craig is homosexual and has AIDS, he will go directly to Hell.

Harold calls his priest (me) and relates the story. I immediately call Craig's parents and reassure them about Craig's salvation. My appeal seems to work. (To be sure of his salvation I do not wait, but administer extreme unction now.)

Craig's parents arrive in extremis but decline to visit him. I spend several hours trying to convince them of the importance of reconciliation before death. Craig is sinking fast; his parents, mercifully for all concerned, visit him as he lay dying.

It's Monday, and the funeral is not until Friday. I spend several hours each day talking with the parents. At the funeral, Craig's parents 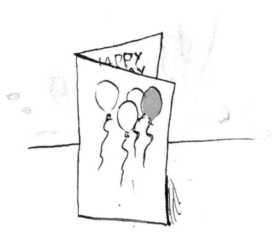 courageously tell the congregation that their son was gay and died, at age 31, of AIDS. A cleansing confession.

The funeral is on my birthday, and for years after, every one of my birthdays is greeted by a memento birthday card from Craig's mother.

(RR)

I DIED FROM AIDS (NOT)

Exhaustion. That word best describes the impact on public health workers confronting the AIDS epidemic in its early days. Not only is this new epidemic mysterious, but efforts to control this rapidly-fatal syndrome are mired in acerbic political and ideological space. Stress levels are high everywhere, not only in the populations deeply affected by the AIDS burden, but also with the employees in health departments charged with stemming its propagation. "Relentless" accurately describes the pressure felt by many of these infectious diseases workers who are, in addition, hounded by the press at any hour of the day or day of the week.

Humor is great medicine. And so the day comes when Bob, a health department disease sleuth, declares: "You don't get bored, just burned out. I'm thinking of making a T-shirt that reads:

"I DIED FROM AIDS

AND I DIDN'T EVEN HAVE IT." [6]

(**NS, RK**[7])

---

[6] Bob's quote was taken from *LIFE* magazine: Healy, Rita. "The AIDS Tracers". *LIFE,* October 1987: 52–55.

[7] Dedicated to the memory of Bob Kellner (1948–2003).

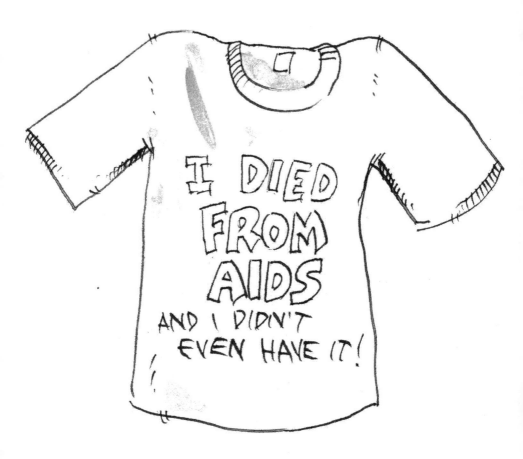

When Death is not a Statistic

This afternoon I receive a call from a friend of long ago, Tim. He is the ex-boyfriend of a former, long-term coworker in our AIDS control program, Doug. The pleasure of hearing his voice again after all these years turns to pain upon learning that Doug has just died of AIDS. Would I come to his memorial service? Looking forward to reconnecting with Tim and to seeing familiar faces, I accept and immediately place a call to yet another AIDS coworker, Greg.

Greg's roommate answers the phone but wants to know how well I know him, telegraphing his wariness of a woman asking to speak to his lover. He no sooner accepts my explanation of our long ago professional relationship than he reveals that Greg died of AIDS yesterday, and that a memorial service is being arranged.

Talk about a lightning fast one-two punch! Floors me.

Overwhelmed with grief, I leave the office and head home, crying all the way. Crying not simply for their suffering and loss, but also in gratitude for all the personal and professional energy they invested in the fight against AIDS.

There are times in every public health worker's life when she truly learns that death is more than yet another statistic.

(NS)

PART IV: HIV / AIDS

Part V: Prostitution

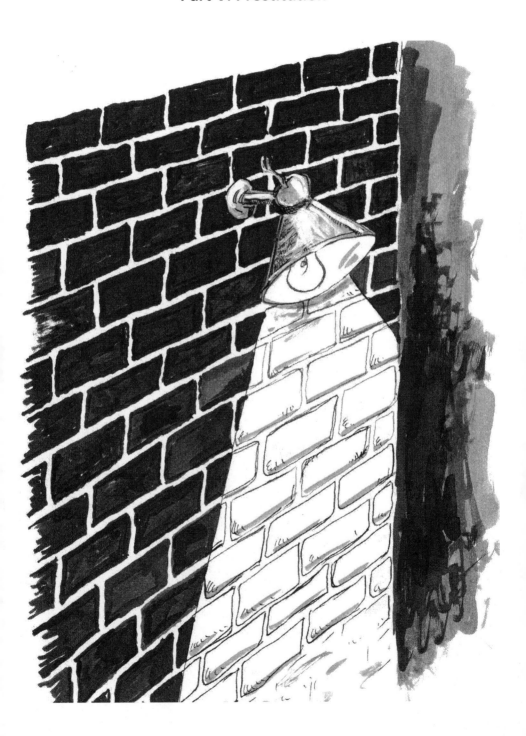

La Prostitution Oblige

We're waiting impatiently for its arrival. It's now the spring of 1985, and a reliable test for HIV is finally becoming available. Because this virus is transmitted by specific sexual and drug using behaviors, it makes sense to screen populations known to engage in them. In our city, one such population consists of street prostitutes. Fortunately, most of these women are well-known to our staff in the VD clinic, and vice-versa.

Treatment for this rapidly fatal infection is seemingly years down the road. This realization, coupled with strong fears that the HIV-infected will be discriminated against, leads public health authorities to discourage high-risk people from being tested. Not us. We feel that it's better for individuals to know than to pretend "it couldn't happen to me" and for the community to know where HIV infections are concentrated.

We are told by the HIV control professionals at both State and Federal levels that prostitutes are not likely to accept testing. Because this is an assertion I suspect is based on opinion rather than field experience, I decide to ask prostitutes on the stroll (where they work) if they would be willing to be tested for HIV. The very first response is: "Of course we should be tested!" As we soon find out, this attitude is widely shared by these women. Expert opinion trumped again!

If Noblesse Oblige is defined as "the inferred responsibility of privileged people to act with generosity and nobility toward those less privileged", then La Prostitution Oblige can be viewed as the inferred responsibility of prostitutes toward possibly harming clients. Me? I see their willingness to be tested for HIV as an act of generosity and nobility.

(JJP)

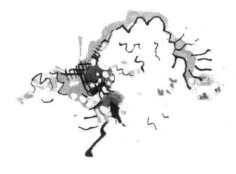

PART V: PROSTITUTION

Trust Indicator

During our four decades of working closely with street prostitutes, we at the health department's VD clinic have earned both their trust and a national reputation for how to work collegially with these (often endearing) outlaws. As a consequence, I'm sometimes asked to supply anecdotes to support claims of mutual trust. Here's one.

Sandra is a circuit prostitute treated in our clinic for secondary (the rash stage) syphilis who I, as contact tracer, interview for sexual partner information. She names mostly her regular, and a few of her casual, local customers. Because she services "johns" in Rocky Mountain states and areas directly north, she soon finds herself in a rural private physician's office in Canada for our recommended periodic VD check-up. She's told she has a positive blood test and needs treatment. She tells the physician that she's recently been treated for syphilis and that, based on what she's told in our clinic, "the blood test probably hasn't yet had time to return to negative".

When the physician tells her she must be re-treated in any case, Sandra calls me to seek, in her words, "trustworthy advice". My advice is to wait two weeks and repeat the blood test; if the numerical value rises two or more intervals from the baseline value, then the physician's caution is warranted. If it stays the same or, likelier, declines, then no treatment is needed.

Sandra appreciates not having to suffer two probably unnecessary penicillin shots in her derrière—and gratefully tells me so the next time we meet. And the beat goes on.

(HLR)

Time is Money

As a private dermatologist moonlighting in the health department's VD clinic one night a week, I'm rapidly improving at the pelvic examination craft. It takes weeks before I pay sufficient attention to notice that a few women undress in unorthodox fashion.

Whereas most women remove whatever underwear, panties, panty hose, and shoes they come in with, arranging these items on a chair, a few women leave them wrapped around one ankle. Curiosity prompts me to ask my nurse, knowing that being a woman and having worked in VD clinic for decades, she surely can explain it. "They're working girls, Doctor, street prostitutes who 'turn-over' clients fast and need to undress and dress again as quickly as possible."

After all, time is money.

(GSM)

Massage Parlor Dry Skin

Annette is a ravishing young woman who works in a local massage parlor. She's in clinic today for a routine VD check-up, an occupational necessity. Her only symptom is "dry, itchy skin all over". Being a dermatologist, I'm delighted to recommend my favorite moisturizing lotion, to be applied after showering. To get a sense for how much she'll need, I ask Annette how often she showers: "Once a day". This surprises me because, even though we live in a state with very low humidity, her skin is much drier than expected. On further questioning, she confesses that, about half a dozen times a day, she joins her clients in the hot tub, for sexual purposes.

Problem solved: treat massage parlor dry skin with moisturizing lotion after every hot tub exposure.

(GSM)

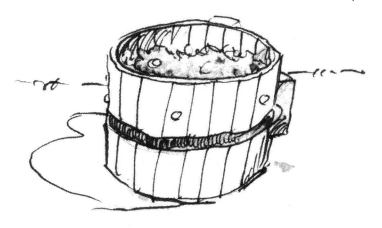

When Irons Fly

Jacqueline is an upscale hotel prostitute. Her nickname is "The Dish" and, as implied by this sobriquet, she's drop-dead gorgeous, with a personality to match. (These attributes are, I suspect, why she's never been arrested for solicitation.)

This evening she's in VD clinic for her routine monthly check-up and, knowing that I'm a dermatologist asks if, after the pelvic examination, I would mind examining a spot on her breast. Of course. She lifts her blouse to expose her left breast, revealing a now crusting triangular red spot.

PART V: PROSTITUTION

Although it looks like the *Star Trek* emblem, I recognize it as a healing second-degree burn.

Curious, I ask what happened. She tells me that about a week ago, while ironing a blouse, her cat suddenly jumps on the board, sending the cradled iron sailing upward, flipping over and hitting her on her breast. Ouch! Not a pretty owie.

Wanting to look your best for your job is good; ironing while naked to achieve this aim is bad (especially if you own a high-jumping cat).

(GSM)

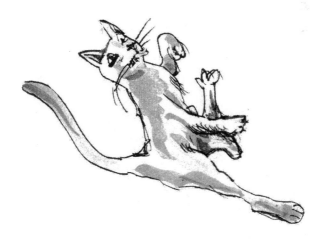

My First and Last

Wednesday night is my favorite of the three VD clinic sessions we offer weekly, and the one most likely to be attended by local prostitutes. Being open between 7pm and 10pm, it's after dinner and just before they hit the streets to solicit "johns".

Rebecca is an attractive rinsed-out blonde in her late twenties who started selling her body from upscale hotel lobbies ten years earlier. Because her girlish good looks are fading, she increasingly sells her charms using a less desirable marketplace: the street.

Unlike many prostitutes, she enjoys her craft, taking pride in both her appearance and professional skills. She coquettishly promotes herself using the acronym V.I.P. (yes, even on her business card, fully spelled out!). In this case, the "P" refers to her *belle chose*, differing from the word "hussy" by only this initial letter.

She's now entering my office, as she regularly does for her customary VD checkup. This time she's beaming, literally bursting with pride. She suddenly

PART V: PROSTITUTION

lifts her braless top to show me her new headlights, as she refers to the outcome of her breast augmentation procedure. Noting my (admittedly mild) embarrassment, she courteously covers herself.

My office colleague, whose back is (regrettably, he later confesses) turned during this flashing encounter, tells me that he had heard of this procedure (relatively new at the time) but has, like me, not known anyone who has undergone it.

It's my first, and last, flashing episode.

(JJP, CP)

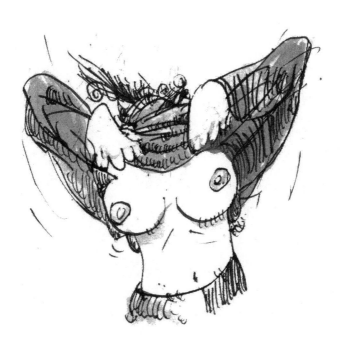

Deep Throat Transmission

Amelia and Kendrick are sitting with me in my office while my nurse prepares the examination room. Amelia is a street prostitute; Kendrick, her pimp; and I'm the physician in this health department VD clinic.

I always enjoy spending time with our prostitutes, making small talk and answering questions. Today, Amelia wants to know why she always has to have a throat culture, a procedure she finds both unnecessary and (especially) uncomfortable, because it makes her gag. I explain that the test looks for infections like gonorrhea and chlamydia. Again, she persists in asking why, and I reiterate that VD is commonly found in the throat of prostitutes, seeing as that they are often asked to give oral sex. Hearing that, Amelia suddenly pivots in her chair and punches Kendrick in the arm, exclaiming: "You told me that it couldn't happen—that it dies when exposed to air". End of misinformation.

As word travels quickly among street prostitutes, it's now seldom that one of our working girls complains about throat culture tests or is misinformed about deep throat VD transmission.

(GSM)

On Death's Door

Victoria is a street prostitute addicted to pain pills, which she regularly buys on the street. Tonight she's in our VD clinic complaining of pain in her lower abdomen. When I examine her, given the pronounced pain on palpation, I suspect pregnancy in her right Fallopian tube and order a pregnancy test, which right away comes back positive. Even though it's already 8pm, I call a gynecologist colleague who agrees to see her soon at the hospital next door.

When I follow up the next day, the gynecologist tells me that Victoria didn't show up until midnight, having gone back on the street to solicit customers and to buy more pain pills. Wheeled into surgery, Lady Luck is on her side because, as he explains, the moment he opens her abdomen the blocked Fallopian tube "popped right up and burst".

Had she waited longer, she would have bled to death.

(GSM)

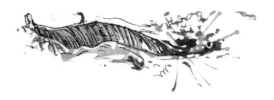

The Condom Curtain

Alicia, a seasoned prostitute, insists on customers "suiting up" for each sexual act—oral, vaginal, or anal. In this Age of AIDS, this is unsurprising. Yet it's only unsurprising, because I interpret her insistence using my values as VD control officer: condoms are an effective barrier to both the acquisition and transmission of sexually transmissible microbes. Good strategy for both of our occupations.

As I compliment her for her contribution to VD control, Alicia duly corrects me: "I don't use condoms to stop venereal disease, but to remain faithful to my man". Puzzled, I ask what she means. She explains that condoms provide a physical barrier to true intimacy—something she reserves for her pimp—not to mention that condoms prevent sperm from entering her body. Doing sex otherwise would be too personal which is also, she tells me, why she never kisses customers.

Is there a better way for a working girl to disassociate sex from love other than hiding behind the condom curtain?

(**JJP**)

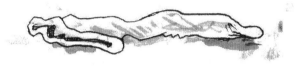

Barbed and Wired

Because she's a street prostitute, Marilyn comes in for a sexually transmitted diseases check-up at least bimonthly. In fact, she holds the record for most number of visits ever by any person, male or female, in our VD clinic. Regrettably she's hopelessly drug- and alcohol-addicted, which is the principal reason her life is chaotic and, above all, dangerous. I know that it's not unusual for some of her more mentally-deranged customers to abuse her.

As I see her walking into the clinic waiting room today I'm delighted to note she's sober, although clearly bearing a pained expression. Before I can greet her she lifts her braless sweater—right in front of about two dozen seated (and startled) patients—to show her profoundly lacerated breasts. Noticing that the deep lacerations are infected, I ask why she waits such an apparently long time to seek medical attention. She doesn't reply, but I suspect that being constantly under the influence of drugs and alcohol prevents her from making good decisions. Long experience confirms that bad things occur when she's "wired". Perhaps, I speculate, she's too embarrassed to come in.

Now, to the $64,000 question: how did this happen? She relates that a trick takes her home, overpowers her (not difficult to do when she's drugged), and ties her up tightly with wire—barbed wire. Sadist sex follows, in all orifices. This is the Nth instance of abuse by some mentally unstable trick, and it pains me to realize that, horrible as many abusive episodes are, this particularly brutal one won't be the last. The hundreds of hours of professional mental health counseling our health department's Drug & Alcohol Program provide over many, many years have sadly not had the desired results.

Marilyn, wired and barbed during decades of alcohol and drug abuse, is 48 when she dies a few years later, of liver failure.

(HPZ)

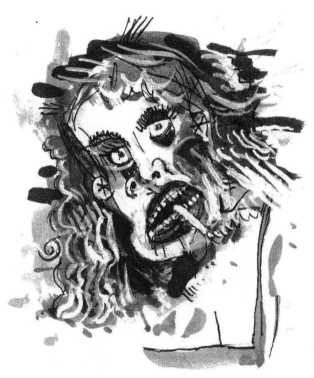

May I Watch?

Cheryl, a veteran street prostitute, is an alcohol- and heroin-addicted injecting drug user so tired of her life that she wants to die. She tells me: "If I have to suck one more cock, I'll puke." She has thought of suicide several times and will again in the future. It's not a thought that goes away even when she's sober and detoxed. She's been "clean" several times, a consequence of the abstinence of incarceration. Once freed, she immediately resumes her ride on the hellbound alcohol and drug train she tells me she can't control. Her mother, a respected local insurance agent who becomes my long-term acquaintance, confirms Cheryl's history. She's heartbroken.

I meet Cheryl in my VD clinic a year or two after she enters prostitution at age 17, referred by the police for mandatory VD testing. During the 18 years that she attends for periodic VD testing, she is afforded professional counseling, primarily in the Drug & Alcohol Prevention Clinic next door. Her reckless sexual, drug use, and driving behaviors, each of which seems to me to be a platform for suicide, continue despite long-term, empathic counseling. Not even her young daughter's presence and love attenuates her self-destructive bent. (That daughter, bright like both her mother and the grandmother who is raising her, eventually graduates from an excellent liberal arts college in Colorado.)

During a period of about a dozen years, she often threatens suicide. She calls me four times, always in the wee hours of the night. Each time I talk her down and drive to her location. The fourth time, exasperated (enough is enough), I ask for permission to come over and watch her do it. Familiar with my impish sense of humor, she parries my outrageous proposal, calls her counselor and goes on with life.

It's the last suicide threat call I receive from Cheryl. We keep in touch for the next 14 years, including through my retirement from public health. She reportedly neither threatens nor tries suicide again, dying at age 50 of drug abuse-related kidney failure.

(JJP)

The Pimp Surrenders

Tyrone secretly tails her car to find out where she's going. Kitty is one of the prostitutes in his stable, and surveillance is one of his periodic tasks. She arrives at our health department VD clinic and, while registering, Tyrone bursts into the waiting room, using his most menacing demeanor and language: "I'm gonna whoop your sorry ass".

I'm a diminutive, middle-aged woman, the clinic nurse practitioner, and I step between them demanding to know what the problem is. Tyrone explains that if she's here, it's because she has venereal disease, which is bad for business. I inform him that if Kitty is infected, it's probably because he infected her (an assessment based on previous experience with our city's pimps) and that he therefore needs to be treated at the same time. He turns his head and mumbles something unintelligible, which I assume is reluctance to be examined. I firmly insist on his registering for clinic.

He meets his match today: Tyrone, the implacable boss of his women, is being bossed around by a resolute female nurse. Tyrone The Pimp surrenders. He registers and is treated. His test, predictably, is positive for gonorrhea.

(HPZ)

Prime Suspect Candidate?

It's my first real job. Although recently certified to teach science to high schoolers, I now realize that I've no desire to teach kids who likely aren't interested in science. Nor am I willing to spend my workdays babysitting them or acting as their jailer.

This job suits my interests and skills, as well as my wish to work for the public good: I'm hired to computerize the health department's VD program records. My first assignment is to create a confidential and safe database to store the program's twenty years of medical and social data on prostitutes working in our region.

Because of space constraints, I work alone in one of the program's only two offices, from late at night until early morning. This graveyard shift not only fits my hermitlike work style, but also affords the quiet I need to concentrate on methodical chart reviews and archived police arrest data. I now have access to a significant amount of information on hundreds of prostitutes, which can easily be examined and retrieved with computerized analytic tools.

My anxiety starts a few months into the job when a rash of deaths among prostitute women, including a few murders, occurs in our city. Many local prostitutes, with whom our VD contact tracers work cooperatively, confess their fears, wondering if some serial killer is responsible for this unusual number of young working girls' deaths. Not only is this my first introduction to the realities of the dangerous world occupied by street prostitutes, but it's also a chilling realization that I might become a suspect. After all, what's keeping me, the lone night owl, and custodian of key data on prostitutes, from using this information for nefarious purposes? Being a new employee who's not well known by coworkers probably qualifies me as a prime suspect candidate.

Ideal job? Just what have I gotten myself into, anyway?

(SQM)

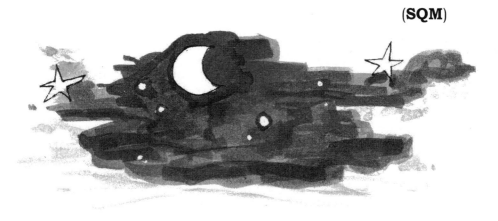

Chocolate, Grape, or Strawberry?

My job as data manager for our health department's study of street prostitutes and injecting drug users frequently finds me working at night. My office is a stone's throw from "the stroll" (where prostitutes solicit). I occasionally leave to get some fresh air and get away from frustrating software debugging tasks. When I do, I grab a bag of flavored (mint for oral sex; chocolate, grape, strawberry and vanilla for sex below the belt, front or back) condoms, as well as little bottles of bleach (to sterilize needles) in case I run into (often drug-addicted) working girls.

Tonight, from barely a block away comes a large woman who, using her rehearsed abrupt demeanor, shrill voice, and confrontational stance yells: "Hey YOU! Yes YOU! I'm talkin' to YOU! I seen you around before. In fact, I seen you around a LOT. But you know what? I ain't never seen you buy no pussy!" To which I reply: "That's because I'm a terrible liar." She looks at me in puzzled amazement. I explain that were I to yield to temptation, my girlfriend would surely find out, grab my privates and whirl me around like David with his slingshot just before felling Goliath. That melts the ice. She dissolves in shrieks of laughter.

I now open my "stroll bag". Her eyes get big: "Oh, you're one of those health department guys. You got any flavored ones?" She's simultaneously yelling for her running partner who magically emerges from around the corner. For the next few minutes they make editorial comments as they fish for their favorites: "No, not the chocolate ones. Do you have strawberry? They're the best…"

Ah, the joys of shopping!

(SQM)

Of Porn Stars and Co-Stars

She's pretty and poised as she sits across from me in my office at the VD clinic. She's here because she has vaginal symptoms, a bit worried that it's VD "because this would involve a lot of people".

I see her two days later for test results, which are positive for both gonorrhea and chlamydia. Taking this news with surprising aplomb, she's eager to tell me about her sexual partners and also about her partners' partners. In all my years as a VD contact tracer, I've never seen anyone so ready to talk. My question is: "Why?"

She and her partners are in the pornographic film industry. She's disappointed that the mandated, frequent VD/HIV testing system failed to detect the very infections it's designed to detect. I tell her that someone got through the normal safeguards, because that person's test specimens may not have been properly collected or tested.

To make things easier, I arrange for group testing and treatment of her co-stars and film crew at a specially-scheduled, closed clinic session.

(PM)

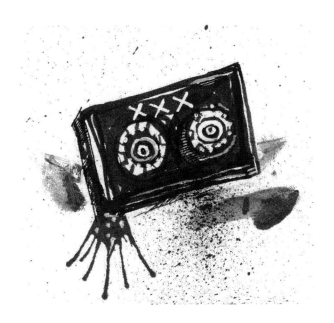

Friend or Foe?

Summer of 1987. It's evening and I'm on my second date with a lady who, six months hence, becomes my second wife. She knows that I moonlight at the VD clinic from my private practice as a dermatologist.

She also knows that I've dated several other women since my divorce.

We're sitting at a gas station in my white Mustang convertible, top down, about a block from the "stroll" (where street prostitutes solicit). Out of the adjacent parking lot runs a young woman with large, pendulous breasts, wearing a skin-tight see-through T-shirt, repeatedly yelling "Hi, Doc!" at me. No sooner does she reach my car that she leans over the passenger side door, leaning her upper body almost in my date's face.

After exchanging a few pleasantries, gassed up, I drive off. That's when my future bride asks: "Is this one of your old girlfriends or one of your clinic patients?" The acid test for continuing our date, I suppose.

(GSM)

For Hire, For Higher

Summer, 1992. I'm in Amsterdam to present a paper about prostitution, drug abuse, and HIV risk at the International AIDS Conference. This is my first oral presentation at a notable scientific meeting and, being inexperienced, am a bit nervous. Time for taking in a little noon fresh air and sunshine by walking this charming city.

I soon see a woman coming down the street who's making eye contact with me. I keep walking, pretending not to notice. She gently accosts me, eyes my outline suggestively and, rolling her "r"s in an unmistakable Scottish brogue says: " I can r-r-really r-r-relax yeh. And even take you higher-r-r." I politely decline, thank her for so refreshingly stroking my ego, explain my presence in Amsterdam, and ask if she would join me for lunch.

We sit at an outdoor café, where I order lunch and black espressos for us. She seems anxious, furtively looking around. It doesn't take me long to realize that she's worried about plainclothes policemen spotting her, for in Amsterdam only state-approved and certified disease-free women working in licensed brothels are permitted to ply their trade. She tells me that things have been tough for her and her 12-year-old son, and that making the rent is a chronic challenge.

Lunch lasts a half hour, during which she periodically hunches down to avoid being spotted. I pay the bill, tip the waitress, and discreetly slip some money her way in appreciation for her company. Surprised, she smiles and sweetly bids me good luck and good-bye. I reciprocate and we part.

The convergence of her offer (for hire... for higher, as it were) and the subject of my presentation is pure irony.

It remains a treasured memory.

(SQM)

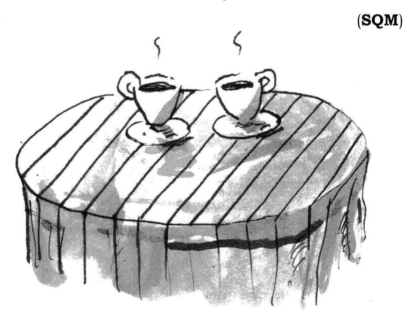

PART V: PROSTITUTION

Part VI: Behind the Scenes

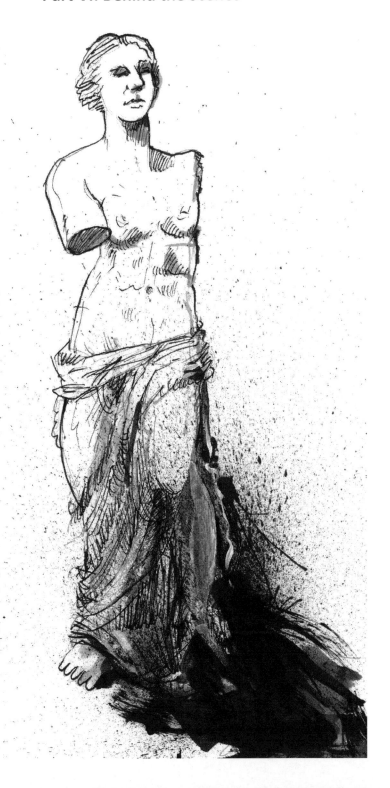

The Day I Dodged the Bullet

It's not unusual for a sexually transmitted diseases contact tracer to be propositioned by a client. A minor occupational hazard, it's easy to avoid.

It's 1983 and Bruce, a gay man in his late thirties, is being treated for syphilis at our local VD clinic. When we meet to discuss his sexual partners I, being a young woman, am relaxed about being propositioned, because I assume his sexual orientation is exclusively homosexual. Imagine my surprise when he tells me that he'd like to have a sexual relationship with me. I tell him that I'm happily married and do not "fool around". Not inclined to settle for "No", he gently, without any coercion in his approach, says: "Oh, I get it, you think I want to do it the way I do it with the others I just told you about: up the behind." Although I know that receptive anal intercourse is the only sexual behavior associated with AIDS, I reply that I'm not thinking that way, and that the reason I decline is that mine is not an open marriage. End of negotiation, which he takes in stride.

Years later, when AIDS is shown to commonly occur in gay men who are diagnosed with syphilis, I realize that I likely dodged this deadly bullet thanks to professional ethics (which I didn't tell him about) and marital fidelity.

(NS)

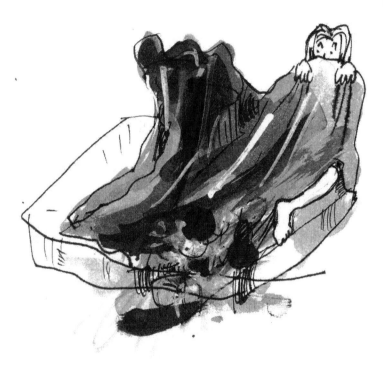

Data Entry Dilemma

As VD program supervisor, the day I dread more than any other actually arrives. It's the first time, and I've no experience other than having cursorily thought about it in the past. It's the day my data entry clerk Barbara, a young woman who's coupled with long-time boyfriend Trevor, sees his full name and locating information on the standard form used for persons exposed to VD, in this case both gonorrhea and chlamydia.

Given that there are two practical jokers on staff, Barbara tries to figure out which by the handwriting (these forms are rarely typewritten), but this handwriting belongs to neither. This form may be for real. Panic. Because contact forms are linked by code with the index patient who names him as a partner, she can now find out who her boyfriend's sexual partner is. And she does. Panic again. Above all, rage—because the other woman is her good friend Jenny.

My job is to calm her and remind her that whatever her adrenal glands tell her to do, she cannot let either Trevor or Jenny know that she knows. Medical confidentiality protects Jenny from being discovered as the information's source the moment she names any sexual partner, and no named sexual partner is entitled to know who names him. Ironclad and time-honored promise. Barbara, crushed and feeling helpless, knows the consequences of betraying confidentiality.

She's crushed again when Trevor tells her that he's infected and may have infected her. Neither relationship, with either Trevor or Jenny, survives this damning proof and pain of cheating hearts.

(**HLR**)

Cretin

She's a bright middle-aged nurse who's not yet sufficiently familiar with our computer database routines. He's the exceptionally-gifted database architect, about fifteen years younger, and not yet sufficiently patient with explaining its workings to mere mortals.

The day comes when her frustration reaches the boiling point. She bursts into my office (I'm the boss) venting her fury as she details her encounter of a few minutes ago with the impatient computer guru, specifically referring to him as a cretin.

As I know his father well, I reach him and express surprise that his computer-geek son was born in Greece. Puzzled, his father tells me that this son was born in New Orleans, not Greece. Puzzled in turn, I explain to him that one of my nurses just called him a cretin, and that my admittedly modest knowledge of modern Mediterranean history places Crete within the Greek polity.

It takes just a second for the pun to sink in. Both father and I explode in laughter.

(JJP, SQM)

Don't Try This at Home

The VD caseworker's most desirable attribute is tolerance. If good-natured live-and-let-live tolerance doesn't come naturally, you must develop it until you become at least professionally nonjudgmental.

I'm a recently-married woman in her late twenties, working as a contact tracer in the health department's VD control program. Presently, I'm interviewing a married man whose sexual partners other than his wife include several prostitutes whose company he genuinely enjoys. He feels sufficiently comfortable revealing graphic details of these extramarital encounters that he finally blurts out: "I wish my wife were as understanding as you!"

I'm now relating this anecdote to my husband who knows full well that such tolerant "understanding" is unlikely ever to apply to our marriage. As he quickly and accurately points out: "he wouldn't have said that if he actually lived with you!"

(**HLR**)

Balls

It takes balls to play tennis. Chasing tennis balls is one of my preferred leisurely pursuits. In real life, I run a VD control program. My seasoned staff has just extinguished a turbocharged epidemic of venereal diseases in crack-cocaine street gangsters and their sexual contacts. It takes more than a year to stop this furious outbreak, no mean feat considering the actors and the stage. The actors are, on one side, young black men just emerging from adolescence and their mostly adolescent and ethnically diverse female sexual contacts and, on the other side, white health department contact tracers, often a decade and a half older than they. The stage is the mean streets occupied by rival gangs.

Oil and water? No.

These outlaw populations may be alienated, but they are not aliens. They prove this by cooperating to stop disease transmission. They identify not only their sexual contacts, but members of other gangs (there are five of them) who, they tell us, might benefit from being tested. Because such cooperation by street gangsters hasn't been reported in the medical literature, I prepare a manuscript intended for the Centers for Disease Control's (CDC) influential medical bulletin. It turns out that the editors do not want the description of this exceptional outbreak to include race/ethnicity or its occurrence in street gangs. (So much for the central tenet of epidemiology: that it's about Person, Place, and Time.)

Compliance with CDC's wishes risks shrouding person-and-place in a fog. Several long-distance conversations between me, who abhors mental fogginess, and CDC officials, who lean to the fogginess of political correctness, produce an acceptable compromise: race/ethnicity is to be removed from the report. But in a subsequent call, CDC insists that "gang" also be expunged from both title and text. This is unacceptable. Knowing my reputation for "ribald humor, sometimes impatient and brusque manner, and occasional short temper", staff members are then not surprised to see me raging down the clinic corridor after this particularly exasperating phone call, declaring: "They can have one testicle, but they are not getting two!"

After further unpleasant CDC brinksmanship, my resolute refusal to back down registers. The manuscript is published with all relevant person (including race/ethnicity) and place details, but only after I threaten to withdraw the manuscript and file a formal complaint about inappropriate medical censorship.

To this day I have two balls in my pockets when I play tennis.

(**JJP**)

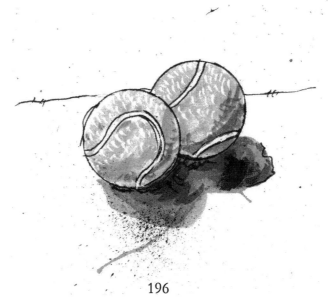

PART VI: BEHIND THE SCENES

Close Encounter of the Embarrassing Kind

It's Friday night, a time when my wife Susan and I grab a bite and go to the movies, having secured a trustworthy babysitter for our young children. Susan, a stay-at-home mom, enjoys the pleasure of going out, and I'm happy to have a break from patients in the VD clinic, my professional home for the past eight years.

I'm well known in my mid-size community, especially among the young, and I not infrequently encounter a patient in public. In almost all cases, when someone recognizes me, s/he does not let on that we're acquainted.

On this particular Friday night, a young couple is crossing the street in a downtown intersection, just as Susan and I are now doing, but from the opposite direction. The young woman's eyes settle on mine and, with a smile, spontaneously exclaims: "Don't I know you from somewhere?"

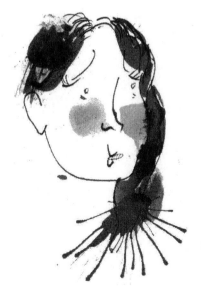

She then immediately corrects herself by saying: "Oooops! No, I don't!"

(**JJP, SBP**)

Would You Ride Me?

It's Halloween and though it's a workday at our health department's central registry for sexually transmitted diseases (where the public is not allowed), employees usually dress in its spirit. Along with their costumes, they bring their *joie de vivre* as do I, along with my impish sense of humor. Although a respectable married woman in her early thirties, I dress as a dominatrix: short-shorts (real short!), fishnet stockings, black boots, fedora hat and, of course, riding crop and handcuffs, with keys on a chain around my wrist.

It's also the day that a renowned epidemiologist from Atlanta's Centers for Disease Control visits our program, for reasons that are not clear to me. This physician and I hit it off immediately, probably because of a shared predilection for impish humor, which explains why he asks: "Wo-Wo-Wo-Would you ride me?" Delighted to comply, I handcuff him, he gets down on all fours, and I simulate whipping his bottom with my riding crop. Kids again!

Was it our playful, devilish sense of humor or my roguish costume that bonded us forever?

(**NS**)

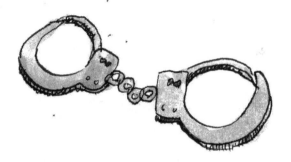

Me and Mr. Jones

Mr. Jones and I both work in venereal disease control in Colorado, about 100 miles apart, and we're both happily married. Every time I talk with him over the phone, which we periodically need to do, he literally makes me sweat. It's a reaction that does not escape my coworkers' notice.

I don't know if it's the sound of his voice, good looks, dry wit, unassuming and gentlemanly demeanor, professional competence, or willingness to collaborate on work projects, but my reaction remains the same every time we connect. Is it due to just one or all of the above? (Oh, and did I mention that he is several years older than I, and that I like older men?)

Whenever Mr. Jones (now "Don") calls, it's usually to check on some routine matter, the domain of clerical staff. Knowing my feelings, these staff members eventually transfer Don's call to me, especially enjoying dramatically and loudly announcing: "I'm transferring Don Jones to you". Moreover, staffers relish watching me slowly and deliberately prepare for (breath control time!)...and then take...and then savor...the call.

Does this composure preparation diminish the sweating? No.

Does Mr. Jones know? Yes, because I eventually tell him.

Do these romantic feelings have a future? No. They simply remain in the delicious realm of fantasy.

(NS)

Abstinence Fails More Often Than Condoms

Part of my job as health department VD control officer is to honor requests from schools to talk to adolescents about sex—specifically about prevention of untoward outcomes, such as unplanned pregnancy and venereal disease. Through the 1960s and 1970s, this turns out to be straightforward: simply provide the scientific facts and let students process the information through their own moral and religious filters.

In blow the conservative moral winds of the 1980s and such presentations now take place in an ideological minefield. Many school administrators respond to public pressure by vocal minorities and encourage conservative values over dispassionate, action-oriented self-defense information. Condoms are viewed negatively, for they "promote sexual adventurism" and "interfere with God's reproductive plans". In several high schools, I'm even asked not to use certain (radioactive?) words, such as abortion and meditation (of all things!) and to emphasize sexual abstinence.

Imposing conservative moral values on adolescents is not what this public official is paid to do (or is comfortable with). Knowing what I know about hormones and adolescents and knowing how difficult it is to delay sexuality much beyond the teen years, I prefer to equip young people with workable, rather than ideological, solutions to prevention.

Why? Because I know that abstinence fails more often than condoms.

(JJP)

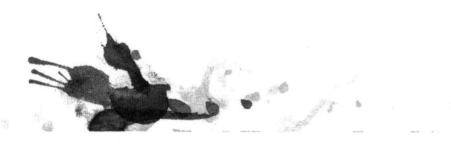

Are You Bigger Than This? If So, Then...

The decade following 1986 is the apogee of the so-called Heterosexual AIDS Scare. Our health department's sexually transmissible diseases (STD) program is constantly being asked to conduct sexual self-defense presentations to heterosexual populations. Male condoms are a principal feature of a menu of recommended defenses, despite considerable resistance offered by people who object to their use for religious or ideological reasons. (Even the Surgeon General of the United States recommends their use.)

The third source of resistance is men, who list several objections, the most frequent of which is "reduced sensitivity" during sex. A legitimate concern. A far less legitimate concern is not uncommonly voiced by male students in local junior, or especially, high schools. "I'm too big for these things" is the stereotypic chortle.

And so I, a young woman in her mid-twenties who works for the STD program, learn to blow up condoms into balloon-like shapes to demonstrate a condom's easy capability to accommodate even giant penises. And at such presentations I look directly into the questioner's eyes and ask: "Are you bigger than this? If so, then..."

Such male braggadocio comments always remind me of my belief in man's infinite capacity for self-deception.

(HLR)

Of Prevention Messages and Teenagers

Today I'm giving a standard talk about sexually transmitted disease prevention to the assembled student body of a local upper-middle-class high school. As usual, I stress taking personal responsibility and making decisions using the cerebral, rather than adrenal, cortex. I provide a broad menu of sexual self-defense choices ranging from abstinence, to delaying sexuality until adulthood, to use of low-risk sexual practices (masturbation, oral sex), to barrier protections, to monogamy. I tell them that they also need to make thoughtful decisions to prevent other harmful (but non-sexual) behaviors.

Being a few minutes before 10am, I conclude this hour-long presentation by enumerating non-sexual but potentially deadly behaviors, such as reckless driving, not wearing a seat belt, smoking cigarettes, and doing street drugs.

I return to my health department office and, mid-afternoon, receive a call from a member of the school staff that a 15-year-old student has been killed. It turns out that, during lunch hour, a group of

PART VI: BEHIND THE SCENES

students was in a jeep at high speed, and the driver failed to negotiate a turn, catapulting the 15-year-old girl, who was not wearing a seat belt, dozens of feet from this jeep.

The teens were on their way to a nearby convenience store to buy cigarettes.

(JJP)

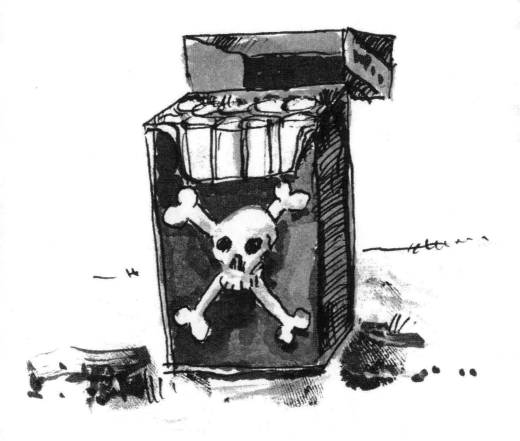

You're Making it Easier for People to Sin

Ours is an internationally recognized sexually transmitted diseases control program. Word of its innovative and empirically-proven strategies reaches the ears of our local government officials who, over coffee and bagels, congratulate our health department team for its VD control achievements. Naturally, this makes us feel proud, immodestly enough.

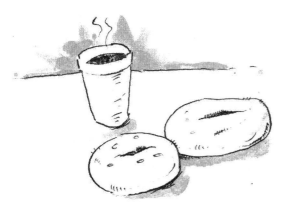

Imagine my surprise when a highly-placed politician discreetly pulls me over to the side and asks: "John, why do you do such a good job cleaning up the community of these diseases? You're only making it easier for people to sin."

I usually assume that people think just like me until startled, by some surprising statement, into realizing that that's not necessarily true. Indeed, until that very moment, it simply never occurs to me that someone could even think such a thought about my life's work.

The end of my (public health career) innocence.

(JJP)

Government Has No Business in the Bedroom

Pierce is a well-known and outspoken member of our community. I'm the well-known and outspoken director of sexually transmissible diseases control in our community. Although he claims to like me ("This isn't about you, John; this is about what you do") he strongly disagrees with using contact tracing as principal tool to interrupt VD transmission. Asking infected people to supply the names and locating information of exposed sexual partners and then contacting them to inform them of potential exposure is, to him, an unnecessary invasion of personal liberty. It's even worse if done at public expense, as is the case here. In his words "Government has no business in the bedroom"

Startled by his view, I ask why. He tells me that infected people should notify their own partners without government acting as an intermediary. His position is unaffected by my explanation that such an approach is "the tried and the untrue": plenty of evidence supports the view that infected patients not only seldom notify their partners but, when notified, partners often fail to follow through for medical care (major reasons: denial, or lack of symptoms, or a cavalier attitude towards health matters). Besides, he assures me: "People who get these diseases deserve them".

The world has an adequate supply of mean-spirited ideologues; Pierce is one of them.

(JJP)

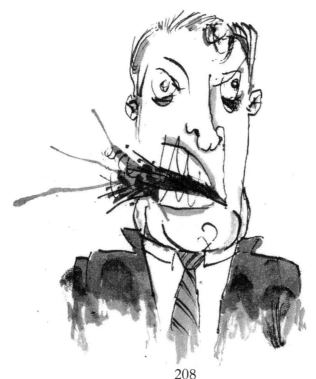

PART VI: BEHIND THE SCENES

Coffee, Tea, Fisting?

Some gay men engage in a sexual practice called fisting, sometimes called handballing or, more crudely, fist-fucking. It consists of inserting a hand into a rectum; once in, fingers are either kept extended or clenched into a fist.

Drawing a sample of blood in the field from a person exposed to syphilis is convenient for both exposed partner and me, a health department contact tracer. Minimal blood-draw training for contact tracers is considered sufficient in the pre-AIDS era. But with the arrival of AIDS contact tracing in the late 1980s, proficiency standards rise, as do precautions to avoid accidental needlesticks. No longer is it satisfactory to simply watch an experienced person draw blood, or to practice on an orange, or to spend a single afternoon drawing bloods in VD clinic. Enter: a newly-designed training machine, featuring a fake arm extended into a tight fist, fake veins, and fake blood. It's mounted on a rolling cart. Virtual reality!

After today's practice session, I see my colleague rolling the cart back to its closet. The fully extended, fisted arm reminds me of a flight attendant pushing a refreshments cart, asking: "Coffee, tea, soft drink?" except that my impish sense of humor audibly edits it to: "Coffee, tea, fisting?"

This now becomes, tongue-in-cheek, the routine announcement to office and venereal disease staff when the cart emerges from its closet.

(**NS**)

Black Sheep of the Family

I'm told there's one in every family: a black sheep. In our respectable and well-behaved family it's my relative Carlos who, in his early teens, joins a local street gang.

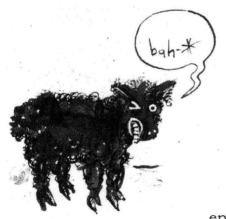

As if this weren't embarrassing enough, he engages in reckless behaviors that soon earn him a place as a patient in the local VD clinic. His first gonorrhea episode occurs at age 15; it's followed by multiple fresh episodes of gonorrhea or chlamydia, transmitted from (and to) multiple and diverse sexual partners, during the ensuing several years. A public health (and personal) embarrassment.

Why stop at two embarrassments: joining a street gang and becoming a venerealaholic? Why not add a third? And so he does, as he visits our health department drug abuse clinic for the first time while entering his twenties. Because drug abuse is a chronic relapsing condition, I know he'll be a frequent visitor in the future.

A few years later, there's a fourth. His newborn child is born drug-addicted.

How does one get off a hell-bound train?

(Anonymous)

Knee-Jerk Reaction

I'm at the International AIDS Conference in Amsterdam, where our health department's HIV Program has a poster presentation titled, in large bolded letters, "Restriction of Personal Behavior: Case Studies on Legal Measures to Protect the Public Health".

It takes little time for self-appointed guardians of AIDS political correctness—members of the group ACT UP, consisting principally of gay activists—to find and vandalize our 5' x 3' poster. They shred it to pieces. So much for tolerance of points of view differing from their own.

Never mind that the poster's content has nothing to do with gay men or their behaviors; its focus is on how to manage prostitutes who recklessly continue to ply their trade, despite being infected with the deadly virus. But why study the poster when you can summarily judge its merits on title alone? Knee-jerk (emphasis on jerk) reaction on the part of these Philistines, who vociferously chant "Stop AIDS! Stop AIDS!" as they march through the poster presentation rooms, convinced that such tactics will somehow achieve that goal.

Anticipating the possibility of such anti-intellectual vandalism, I bring a single duplicate of the poster, which remains unmolested for the rest of the conference.

PART VI: BEHIND THE SCENES

The silver lining? This poster is where I initially meet the woman who, ten years later, becomes my significant other.

(SQM)

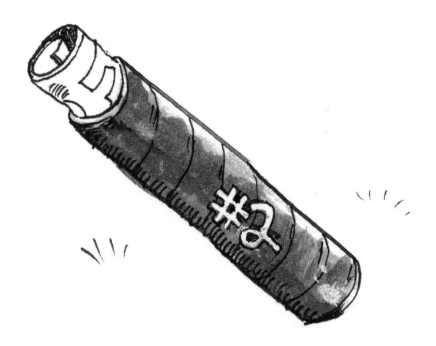

Hairy Tale

It's February of 2000. Don and I are in Vietnam once again after a three-decade absence. This is the fifth day of a seven-day trip, and we travel in a late model sedan, which includes both driver and government-assigned guide/translator.

We're on Route One, which parallels the South China Sea, heading south from the Central Highlands. It's warm and we're thirsty. We decide to quench our thirst at an isolated truck-stop hooch, where refreshments (including women, Don and I subsequently deduce) are available. While driver and guide remain in the car, we approach the thirtyish woman selling cold drinks. Before she can accommodate us, a girl emerges from a back room, looking all of 18 years old (about a third my age). She grabs my arm and begins to stroke its hair, looking in my eyes to gauge my reaction. Suspecting that she may never have touched a hairy arm before, I do not push her hand away. She then lifts my T-shirt and lovingly strokes the hair on my chest, furtively glancing at my eyes. A few seconds later, she grabs my hand and firmly pulls me into the hooch's inner room. Is this girl finding body hair exciting and wants to make love? (Since no upfront money is demanded, I do not suspect prostitution).

Don, a good looker who has barely perceptible body hair, is not approached by either woman. Was this aggressive teen simply waiting until the deed was done before asking for money? Or was she planning to roll me for my wallet once undressed?

It takes a bit of strength to shake free from her grasp and return to the car, where both driver and guide are snickering, trying to keep a straight face. In a minute we are en route on Route One—mystified—and once again heading for Saigon.

(JJP, DEW)

Saving Private Face

Don and I are in Southeast Asia, this time as public health professionals, not as soldiers. Although our HIV conference is in Thailand, we arrange to return, after a three-decade absence, to Vietnam. Hanoi's government has recently opened the country to returning veterans of the "American War", even allowing freedom of travel within its borders. This is appealing, because we both want to revisit the places of significance to us.

We're on our way for a seven-day trip, complete with driver and government assigned guide/translator, in a late model Japanese sedan. The former is about our age (50s), speaks no English and, we surmise, got this cushy job because he fought for the Viet Cong. The latter is a graduate student in economics with good command of English.

After a couple of days of excuses for not taking us to some places of importance to us in the Central Highlands, it suddenly dawns on us that their reluctance may have little to do with selected freedom of travel restrictions. Eureka! This is an Asian country, where saving face is a core value. We suspect they want to spare us the humiliation of seeing the disappearance of the "Welcome Allied Soldiers: We Shall Never Forget You" signs of our day, now replaced by heroic monuments praising the communist victory!

Once Don and I assure them that we are not embarrassed, or ashamed of our defeat, and that seeing these places means more to us than any consideration of reputation, we're driven everywhere we want to go and, indeed, welcomed everywhere we go. We're stunned at the lack of rancor towards

Americans and wonder whether we would have it in our (non-Buddhist) hearts to react similarly had such devastation occurred in our home country.

(JJP, DEW)

IN THE SHADOW OF VENUS

Contributors (Alphabetically, by Initials)

We gratefully acknowledge, and warmly thank, the following for their contributions to this collection of vignettes:

AH   Alex Smart Hinst. Colorado Department of Public Health STD/HIV Programs (1988–1992), Denver CO.

BAD   Beth Dillon, MSW MPH. Colorado Department of Public Health STD/HIV Programs (1982–1987; 1999–2001; 2005–2007), Denver CO.

CP   Christopher I. Pratts, BA. Colorado Springs & Colorado State Health Departments (1973–2000), Colorado Springs & Denver CO.

DDB   Devon D. Brewer, PhD. Alcohol & Drug Abuse Institute, University of Washington (1996–2001), Seattle WA.

DEW   Donald E. Woodhouse, MPA JD. Colorado Springs Health Department STD/HIV Programs (1979–1982; 1987–1996), Colorado Springs CO.

DLG David L. Green, BA. Colorado Springs Health Department STD/HIV Programs (1995-2008), Colorado Springs CO.

GSM Gary S. Markewich, MD. Dermatology & STD Clinic (1973-1975), Fort Carson CO; private dermatology practice & STD clinic physician (1975-1991), Colorado Springs CO.

HLR Helen L. Rogers, BA. Colorado Springs Health Department STD/HIV Programs (1979-2008), Colorado Springs CO.

HPZ Helen P. Zimmerman, BS RN. Colorado Springs Health Department Nursing Section (1959-1972); STD/HIV Programs (1972-2009), Colorado Springs CO.

JJP John J. Potterat, BA. Colorado Springs Health Department, Director: STD/HIV Control Programs (1972-2001). Independent Consultant (2001-present), Colorado Springs CO.

JR Judith U. Reynolds, MD. Colorado Springs Health Department STD/HIV, Drug & Alcohol Abuse Programs (1986–2008), Colorado Springs CO.

LP Lynanne Plummer, BSN RN MPH. Colorado Springs Health Department STD/HIV Programs (1972–1978; 1985–2008), Colorado Springs CO.

NS Nancy E. Spencer, MSPH. Colorado Department of Public Health STD/HIV Programs (1979–2004), Independent Consultant (2005–2007), Denver CO.

PM Pamela Montoya, BA. Colorado Springs Health Department STD/HIV Programs (2001–2003); Colorado Department of Public Health HIV Surveillance (2003–2013), Denver CO.

PZM Patricia Z. Malone, BA. Colorado Springs Health Department STD/HIV Programs (1998–2008), Colorado Springs CO.

RJ Rebecca Jordan, BA. Colorado Department of Public Health STD/HIV Programs (1988–2000; 2006–present), Denver

RK Robert A. ("Bob") Kellner. Colorado Department of Public Health STD/HIV Programs (1980–1988), Pueblo CO.

RR Ronald Raab. Founding Board Member Southern Colorado AIDS Project (1986–1987), Colorado Springs CO.

SBP Susan B. Potterat, BA. Bookseller: Chinook Bookshop (1983–2004); housewife (1969–present), Colorado Springs, CO.

SHS Shana Hurlbutt Sanderson, BSN RN MPH. Colorado Springs Health Department STD/HIV/Hepatitis Programs (2000–2008), Colorado Springs CO.

SKR Sandy K. Rios. Colorado Department of Public Health STD/HIV Programs (1984–1989), Denver CO.

SQM Stephen Q. Muth, BA. Colorado Springs Health Department STD/HIV Programs (1988–2001). Quintus-ential Solutions (2001–present), Colorado Springs CO.

TRE Timothy R. Englert, AB. Colorado Department of Public Health STD/HIV Programs (1974–1979), Durango CO.

TRM Teresa R. Martinez. Colorado Department of Public Health STD/HIV Programs (1998–2017), Denver, Greeley & Pueblo CO.

Title Index

19,000 to 1 Odds	(JJP) 123
Abstinence Fails More Often Than Condoms	(JJP) 201
All in the Family	(TRE) 90
Analomy?	(SQM, Anon) 118
Anatomy Lesson	(HPZ) 24
Apartment #505	(SKR) 86
Are You Bigger Than This? If So, Then...	(HLR) 202
Awakening	(AH) 71
Bad Blood	(HPZ) 96
Balls	(JJP) 194
Barbed and Wired	(HPZ) 171
Beauty and the Beast, The	(SQM, Anon) 37
Birthday Card, The	(RR) 149
Black Sheep of the Family	(Anon) 210
Brothers Who Became Sisters	(NS) 20
Chocolate, Grape, or Strawberry?	(SQM) 178
Close Encounter of the Embarrassing Kind	(JJP, SBP) 197
Coffee, Tea, Fisting?	(NS) 209
Condom Curtain, The	(JJP) 170
Condom Sense, It's	(RR) 117
Cretin	(JJP, SQM) 192
Cruising the Sexual Superhighway	(DDB) 114
Cry the Beloved Mother	(NS) 72
Data Entry Dilemma	(HLR) 190
Day I Dodged the Bullet, The	(NS) 189
Death's Door, On	(GSM) 169
Deep Throat Transmission	(GSM) 168
Definitive Definition	(PZM) 25
Diabla Aquí, La	(PZM) 64
Do You Know Jack, Daniels?	(NS) 82
Don't Try This at Home	(HLR) 193
Double (Triple?) Jeopardy	(NS) 76
Double Whammy	(TRM) 136
Down There	(JJP) 3
Down-Low	(DLG) 128
Every Tom, Dick, and Harry	(DDB) 57
Exit Strategy	(NS) 104
For Hire, For Higher	(SQM) 182
Fourth Man, The	(JJP) 38
Friend or Foe?	(GSM) 181
Geography of Risk, The	(JJP, NS) 85
Get Rid of Smut	(JJP) 119
Gonorrhea Transmission Live (Almost!)	(NS) 63
Gonorrhea, My Eye!	(PM) 11
Goody Two-Shoes	(SQM) 53
Government Has No Business in the Bedroom	(JJP) 207
Gunorrhea Scare	(SQM, Anon) 95
Hairy Tale	(JJP, DEW) 213
Hell Street Blues	(NS) 100
High School Confidential	(HLR) 121
HIV Ending	(JJP) 140
HIV Testing and Murphy('s Law)	(RR) 111
Holly Roller	(BAD) 40
Hoping Against Hope	(DDB) 125
How Much Time Do I Gotta Serve for This?	(NS) 33
Hurricane Mama	(PM) 103
I Didn't Know You Was Gay!	(GSM) 91
I DIED FROM AIDS (NOT)	(NS, RK) 150
I Know How to Make It Hard	(HPZ, JJP) 88
If Asked, Don't Tell	(JJP, LP) 122
In the Swing	(NS, RK) 67
Intersex	(Anon) 27
Interviewing the Dead	(JJP, NS) 146
Intimate Diseases	(HPZ) 112

Investigatory Shot in the Dark, An	(BAD)	47
Irons Fly, When	(GSM)	164
Irresponsible Sex	(Anon)	142
Kealani, And Now	(PM)	147
Knee-Jerk Reaction	(SQM)	211
Likely Story	(BAD)	50
Magnetic	(PZM, DDB)	34
Mankind, Meankind	(NS)	98
Massage Parlor Dry Skin	(GSM)	163
May I Watch?	(JJP)	173
Me and Mr. Jones	(NS)	199
Middle East Meets Midwest	(HPZ)	6
Mobile Front Teeth as Occupational Hazard	(JJP)	18
Mothers, Babies, HIV, and the Future, Of	(AH)	135
Much Better the Second Time Around	(NS, BAD)	43
My First and Last	(JJP, CP)	166
Nasty, Brutish, and Short	(Anon)	132
No Identified Risk Interview	(SKR)	144
No, He Didn't Do It!	(HLR)	94
Not Investigated Rigorously (N.I.R.)	(JJP)	127
Off His Meds	(HPZ, DEW)	138
Pimp Surrenders, The	(HPZ)	175
Porn Stars and Co-Stars, Of	(PM)	180
Prevention Messages and Teenagers, Of	(JJP)	204
Prime Suspect Candidate?	(SQM)	176
Prisoner of Bel-Air, The	(JJP)	84
Prostitution Oblige, La	(JJP)	159
Quality Control	(NS)	77
Queen Guinevere or Lancelot?	(JJP)	92
Rare Beast : Teen AIDS	(DLG)	45
Rebuffed on the Rez	(TRE)	79
Revolving Door Cherie	(DLG)	22
Running the Womens	(DEW)	36
Saving Private Face	(JJP, DEW)	215
Self-Service Surgery, Warts and All	(HPZ)	7
Serious as a Heart Attack	(HPZ)	15
Sexual Boundaries, Anyone?	(Anon)	130
Synagogue Sign Language	(GSM)	9
Taming Hard Rider	(JJP)	12
This Isn't a Lady!	(HPZ, JR)	16
Time is Money	(GSM)	162
Too Good-Looking to be Real	(HPZ)	115
Top to Bottom	(JJP)	46
Traditionalist Christian Sect Welcomes New Member	(PM)	19
Trust Indicator	(HLR)	161
Unto the Next Generation?	(HPZ)	74
Unusual Night Train	(NS, BAD)	65
We Don't Snitch	(NS)	51
What's the Way Out of Here?	(TRM)	102
When Death is not a Statistic	(NS)	153
When Ignorance is a Different Kind of Bliss	(HPZ)	10
Whoever Heard of Gonorrhea of the Elbow?	(NS)	55
Why Did You Wait So Long?	(NS)	75
Why Risk Cutting the Thing You Love Most?	(HPZ)	4
Would You Ride Me?	(NS)	198
You're Making it Easier for People to Sin	(JJP)	206
You're Too Dumb to Charge	(RY)	69

Made in the USA
San Bernardino, CA
04 December 2018